Sameen Ali   Peter Anto Jo
Anthony Chen   John Christy
Avery Kennedy   Asfar Khan
Arnavi Patel   Nasia Sheikh
April Sui   Belinda Tam
Justine Nicole Banszky   Jeremy Steen
Dr. Austin Mardon

What in the World is

Insulin?

GM
PRESS

Typeset and Cover Design by Jedidiah Emms

ISBN: 978-1-77369-234-0
Golden Meteorite Press
103 11919 82 St NW
Edmonton, AB T5B 2W3
www.goldenmeteoritepress.com

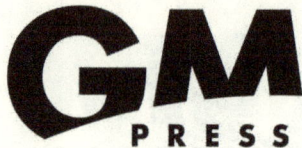

GM
PRESS

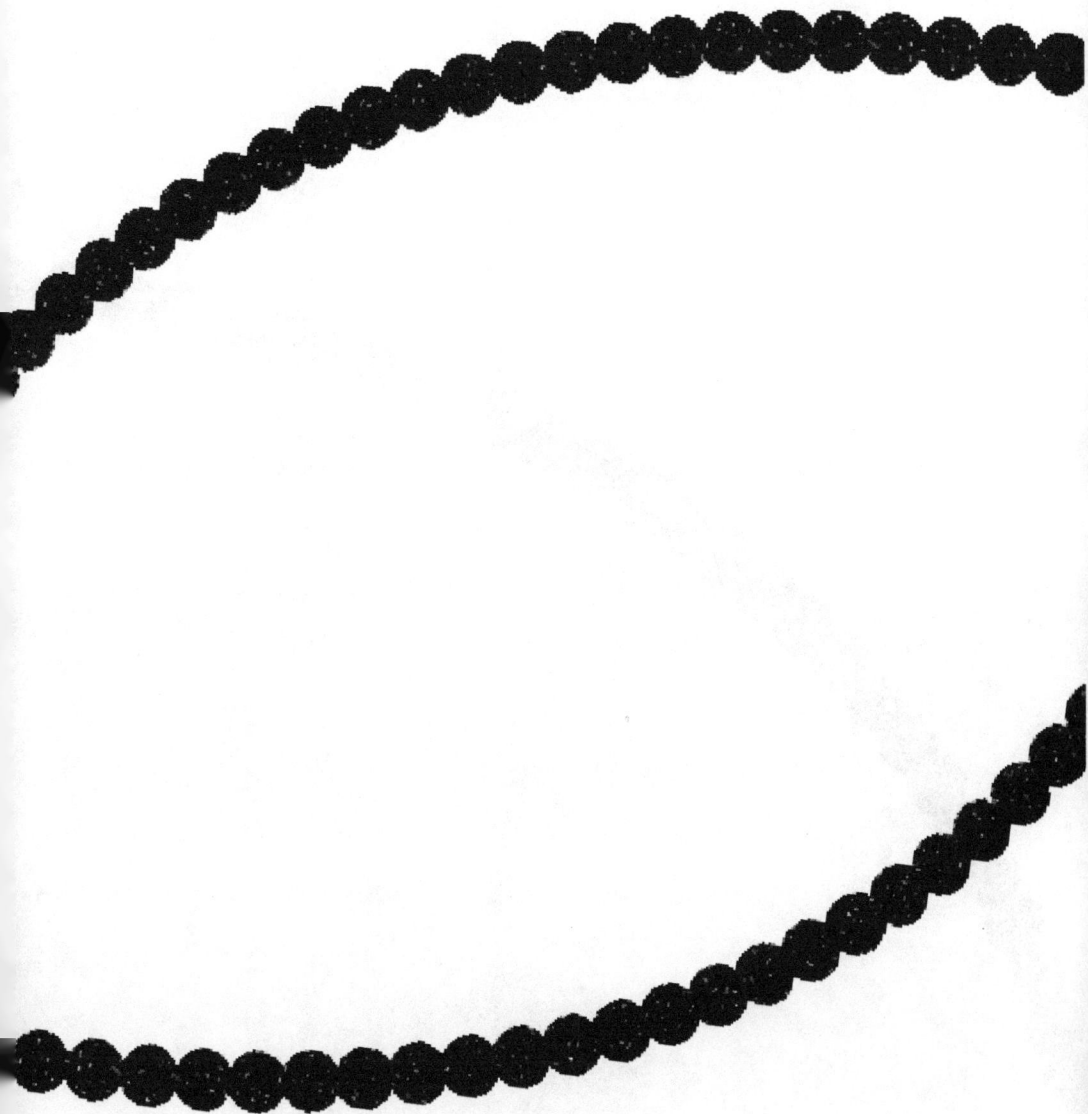

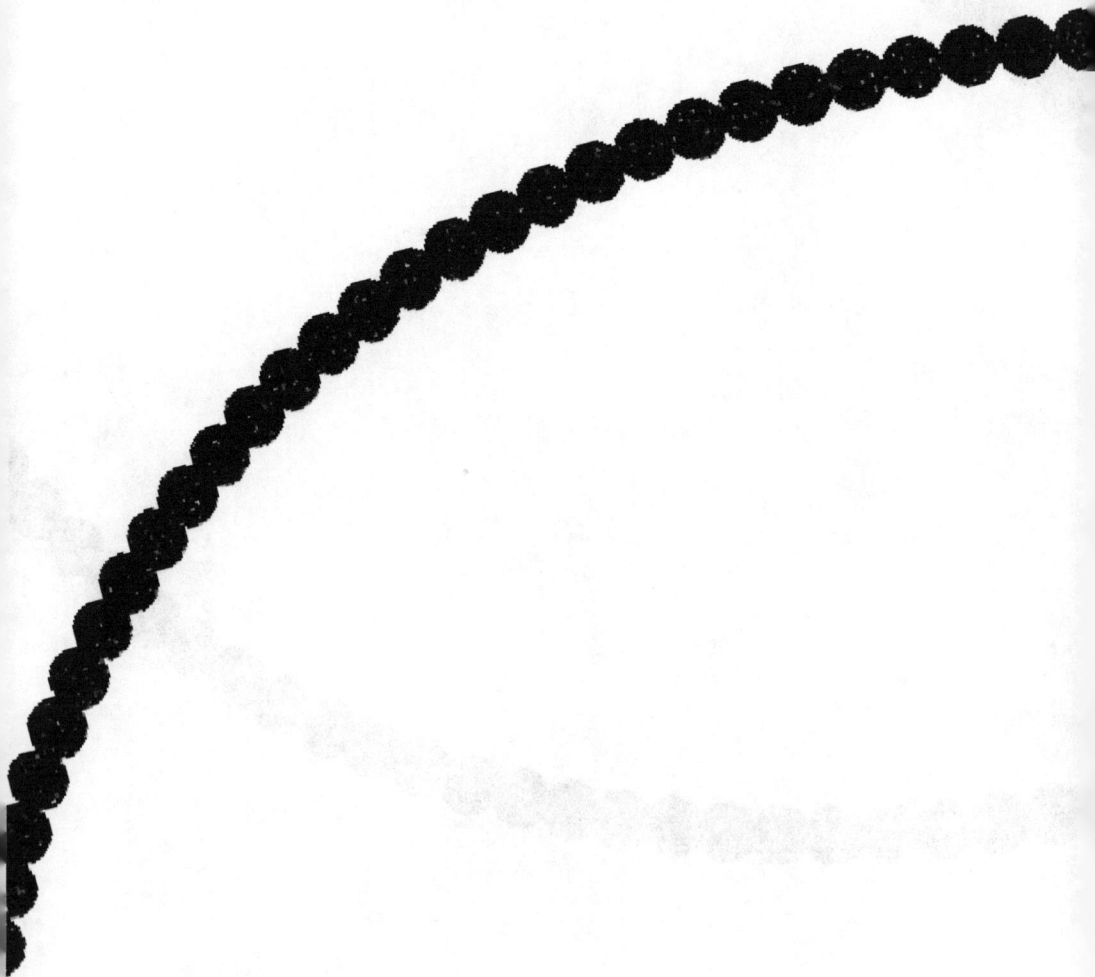

CONTENTS

What in the World is

Insulin?

CHAPTER 1
HISTORICAL BACKGROUND OF INSULIN

Asfar Khan

In 1920, Fredrick G. Banting was a surgeon teaching at Western University in London, Ontario. Banting was scheduled to deliver a presentation to his students on/regarding glucose metabolism. Being unfamiliar with the subject, Banting prepared for this presentation by reading some articles on a late Sunday night. He stumbled across an article called "The Relation of The Islets of Langerhans to Diabetes with Special Reference to Cases of Pancreatic Lithiasis" by Moses Barron. Upon further inspection , Banting came to an epiphany and scrambled to jot down his ideas. In a notebook, Banting wrote, "Diabetes ligate pancreatic ducts of dogs. Keep dogs alive till acini degenerate leaving islets. Try to isolate the internal secretion of these to relieve glycosuria"(1). Soon after, Banting approached James J.R. Macleod, an Associate Dean at the time at the University of Toronto, and an expert in glucose metabolism. Banting explained his hypothesis regarding extracting pancreatic secretions to treat diabetes. Macleod was also the director of the University of Toronto's physiology lab at the time. When approached by Banting, Macleod was at first skeptical of the idea as prior experiments had failed in the past, and Banting did not come from a background in endocrinology. However, although reluctant, Macleod offered Banting his laboratory facilities, and assigned Charles H. Best to Banting, to offer a helping hand. Banting and Best designed a set of experiments using dogs. Their experiments began in May 1921, where the two performed a pancreatectomy on their dog models (1). This meant that the pancreases of the dogs would be removed, which would, in turn, cause the dogs to have diabetes. They then removed the pancreatic ducts, thus preventing the release of any insulin, and harvested the secretions from the ducts. The researchers found evidence that the secretions from the pancreatic ducts resulted in a reduction in blood glucose levels od diabetic dogs (1). Macleod, Banting, and Best were then joined by James B. Collip, who was a biochemist from the University of Alberta visiting the University of Toronto, as he had expressed interest in pancreatic studies . However, although they had found evidence for diabetic therapy through their work, their research received criticism as they had a lack of data surrounding the side effects of their secretions (1).

In 1922, clinicians at the Toronto General Hospital injected a 14-year old diabetic patient with 15mL of the pancreatic secretion created by Banting and his fellow researchers (1). However, the administration of the pancreatic secretions led to little success. A few weeks later, the researchers formed a new set of pancreatic secretions to administer to the patient. The new secretions were formed by James B. Collip who employed a different method to isolate the pancreatic extracts. When administered to the patient, this time the patient responded successfully, showing a significant drop in blood glucose levels. This was the first time in history that evidence for treating diabetes successfully had been found. The group of researchers submitted their findings to the Association of American Physicians during a conference in Washington in 1922 (1). It was then decided that this pancreatic secretion would be called "Insulin" (1). The findings were groundbreaking, and proved a significant advancement for modern medicine. The researchers were met with a standing ovation, and 18 months later were awarded the Nobel Prize in Physiology and Medicine(1).

The development of insulin progressed further in 1922 when the Canadian researchers joined forces with Eli Lilly and Company of Indiana, a reputable company that had expressed interest in the work of the researchers (2). They combined forces as it was difficult for the Canadian researchers to isolate insulin from the pancreatic secretions without contaminating it. And by the summer of 1922, insulin production was underway and being shipped to Toronto for testing. The production of insulin was further ramped up in the fall when chemists at Eli Lilly and Company discovered a method for producing large quantities of insulin through isoelectric precipitation(2). On the other side of the globe, August Krogh and H.C. Hagedorn began producing insulin in Copenhagen in 1923 (2). Krogh had discovered insulin during a trip to Toronto and was eager to treat his wife's diabetes. They began producing insulin at their Nordisk Insulin Laboratory. By the end of 1923, insulin was being used commercially to treat diabetic individuals in western countries (2). The two major producers were Eli Lilly and Company of Indiana, and a subsidiary of Nordisk Insulin Laboratory called Novo (2).

Despite mass production of insulin being well underway, there were still problems that remained. The effects of the insulin obtained through current methods were short-acting. The insulin only lasted about 6 hours, and eventually, the reduced blood glucose levels subsided (2). There was a need for a longer-acting or slow-release insulin that would have long-lasting effects that would counteract hyperglycemia. Researchers at the Nordisk Insulin Laboratory (B.N Jensen, N.N. Krarup, and J. Wodstrup) discovered a method to produce longer-lasting insulin in 1936(2). This was done by combining insulin with a protein known as "protamine" (2). This would allow the insulin to be slowly absorbed, expanding the efficacy time of insulin (2). In 1939, further advancements in insulin were made by researcher David Aylmen Scott, in Toronto (2). Scott created protamine zinc insulin whose blood glucose reducing effects lasted up to 48hours (2). This was almost eight times the duration of the original form of insulin, signifying that drastic improvement of insulin in just under two decades of research (2).

In 1951 the development of insulin further progressed through the introduction of amorphous 'lente' insulins (2). In Denmark, Knud Hallas-Møller, Thorvald, Harald Pedersen, and Jörgen Schlichtkrull, used a new method that combined re-crystallization of traditional insulin and chromatographic procedures and produced a slow release insulin tat was also protamine-free zinc (2)

In 1955, British biochemist Frederick Sanger succeeded in fully sequencing a form of bovine insulin and determined its exact composition in terms of amino acid structure (2). This led to Sanger winning the Nobel for Chemistry in 1958 for his breakthrough. Later in 1964, biochemist, and leader in protein X-ray crystallography, Dorothy Mary Crowfoot-Hodgkin was able to discover the physical structure of insulin (2). As a result, Crowfoot-Hodgkin was awarded the Nobel Prize in Chemistry (2). It was also between 1963 and 1965 that countries across the world (i.e. China, Germany) were able to start synthesizing their own insulin as well (2). Insulin's discovery soon stirred various other discoveries. C.W.A. Kimbell discovered glucagon, a hormone produced by the alpha cells of the Langerhans Islands, with hyperglycemic action, opposed to that of insulin. In 1973, Roger Guillemin discovered somatostatin, another protein polypeptide that was capable of reducing the hyperglycemia in insulin-free diabetes (2).

In 1974, chromatographic purification techniques allowed for the production of purified animal insulin(2). Before this, porcine and bovine insulins would often result in antibody allergies(2). However, with insulin purification techniques improved, there was no significant difference between the purity of animal and human insulins. Subsequently, human insulin was produced using the recombinant DNA technique(2). In 1975, fully synthetic insulin was synthesized in the laboratories of Ciba-Geigy in Basel(2). In a clinical trial conducted at the time, six diabetic patients were treated with synthetic insulin for up to two weeks and It was noted in the article that 2 patients experienced more sudden hypoglycemic events than with animal insulin, but apart from that, the synthetic insulin was well tolerated(2). Charles H. Best, one of the original researchers who discovered insulin, personally commented on this step in the evolution of insulin. Best stated in a personal letter "Dear Dr. Teuscher – I have received your letter and the enclosures. I congratulate your group on the first clinical use of synthetic human insulin. With regards, sincerely – Charles H. Best"(2).

In 1978, scientists from the biotechnology company Genentech in San Francisco, using a combination of genetic techniques, used the plasmids of E. coli bacteria and successfully produced insulin with the same amino acid sequence as seen in humans(2). In 1980, the recombinant DNA 'human' insulin was first tested on 17 non-diabetic volunteers in England(2). Through the experiment, the investigators found that 'human' insulin was slightly more potent than porcine insulin at the low dose, and slightly less so at higher doses. This discovery led to a race to mass-produce 'human' insulin using genetic technology. The race to mass-produce 'human' insulin using genetic technology was eventually won by Eli Lilly in 1982. This resulted in the wide availability of 'human' insulin for the masses. The FDA had approved Humulin R and Humulin N for the US market, which Eli Lilly claimed was identical to human insulin, and this, the best form of insulin therapy to date(2). Overseas, Novo produced semi-synthetic insulins Actrapid HM and Monotard HM, which was also claimed to be the best form of insulin therapy possible(2). As we fell into the 1980s and 1990's, insulin analogs were produced, which were genetically modified forms of insulin that had a slightly altered amino acid sequence. These alterations were done to optimize insulin absorption, distribution, metabolism, and excretion within the human body. In 1996, Eli Lilly introduced the first type of short-acting analog insulin lispro under the brand name Humalog(2). This was followed by aspart, another analog which was approved and released in 2000, and then further down the line glulisine, which was approved and released in 2004(2).

In 2006, Pfizer and Sanofi-Aventis developed a needle-free form of insulin, Exubera. Exubera was an inhaled insulin (2). Pfizer partnered with Nektar to develop an aerosolized form of dry powder insulin that was able to impact human alveoli. This new form of inhaled insulin had a lower bioavailability but was as effective in controlling glucose levels as injectable insulin (2). However, the product proved bulky to use and did not offer any advantage over other short-acting insulin analogs. Therefore, Exubera was removed from the market within a couple of years.

Presently, there are several different types of insulin being offered on the market. Rapid-acting insulin, short-acting insulin, intermediate/long acting insulin and a combination of the different types. Rapid-acting insulin operates over a very short period of time, and works very quickly. Individuals often take this form of insulin right at the start of a meal, as it quickly drops blood glucose levels for a short period of time. This may prevent severe drops in blood sugar in the middle of the night. Short-acting insulin is often used 30-60 minutes before a meal, and takes effect and wears off faster than long-acting insulin. Long-acting insulin contains buffers which slows down the release and allows the effect to be over a long period of time. Finally, a mixture can be created of both rapid or short-acting insulin and long acting insulin which would result in a peak and then a longer duration of effects.

All in all, the development of insulin has progressed significantly over the last century, and has been a forefront of medical advancement. With new advancements and insulin analogs, the burden of daily diabetic care has significantly been reduced. Using long-acting insulin, the amount of insulin injections required have drastically decreased, and this has reduced the risk of hypoglycemia. With short-acting insulins, a convenience has been offered by reducing the need for planning around meal times. In recent years, further developments have been made with the creation of an artificial pancreas. The University of Cambridge, , developed an artificial pancreas in 2013 that was connected to a glucose meter (2). The device continuously measured blood glucose levels, and is also connected to an insulin pump (2). This way, the artificial pancreas will sense an increase in glucose levels and automatically dispense a dose of insulin accordingly (2).

SUMMARY OF TIMELINE

- 1921: Fredrick Banting and Charles Best conduct an experiment to remove the pancreas from a dog, and transfer its contents to a diabetic do, relieving the dog of its diabetic symptoms. They call this pancreatic extract "insulin".
- 1922: 14-year old Leonard Thompson, a type-1 diabetic is the first human subject to receive insulin.
- 1923: Banting and Macleod receive the Nobel Prize in Medicine for their profound discovery
- 1936: Hans C. Hagedorn discovers protamine-insulin which can prolong the effects of insulin
- 1950: Novo Nordisk, a pharmaceutical company based out of Copenhagen create an insulin with an intermediate acting effect

- 1955: Fredrick Sanger discovered the human gene that codes insulin, of which he receives a Nobel Prize.
- 1963: Scientists figure out how to manufacture insulin artificially through genetic technology using Sanger's work.
- 1978: Genetech streamlines the method used to create artificial insulin using DNA recombinant technology.
- 1982: Human insulin (artificial insulin) fills the market, and is much better than animal based insulin.
- 1996: Eli Lilly launches Humalog, a short acting artificial insulin
- 2000+: Modified forms of insulin are released

HISTORY OF INSULIN PRICING

When insulin was discovered back in 1921, Banting, Best, and Collip all had their names attached to the patent awarded in 1923 in their method to make insulin. When they were ready to turn in their patent to allow for the production of insulin, they agreed to only receive $1 each in compensation (3). That $1 was the equivalent of $14 in today's time. It was during this time when the University of Toronto had granted Eli Lilly the right to make insulin, royalty-free, and also offered them the freedom to improve upon the original method/formula and patent anything that they discovered (3). However, come 1941, Eli Lilly and other pharmaceutical companies were being accused of antitrust violations and overcharging for insulin. An article in the Chicago Daily Tribune was released on April 1, 1941, with the headline "Three Drug Firms Indicted by the US: Eli Lilly Is Proud of Insulin Work" (3). The article reported that the companies (Eli Lilly, Sharp & Dohme, and E.R. Squibb & Sons) were indicted for conspiring to unlawfully bring about non-competitive prices of insulin so as to prevent normal competition of sale of the drug. This act violated the Sherman antitrust act,legislation that prevents anti-competitive business practices, and monopolies) (3). As a result, all three companies received fines of $5,000 each, and their leaders faced individual $1500 charges for price-fixing (3).

Since the first analog of insulin was approved, the prices of insulin have gone up steadily. Within the last decade, prices have increased at least 300%, with one vial of insulin costing between $300-$1000 in the US (3). This is because the US has taken a free-market approach to pharmaceutical companies, as opposed to a single-payer system similar to overseas. This means that pharmaceutical companies negotiate privately with private insurance companies over drug prices, giving the pharmaceutical companies more leverage (3). Another reason this exists is that there is no form of generic insulin. Insulin manufacturers have made significant progress in the improvement of insulin products, which has allowed them to stay patent-protected.

CHAPTER 2
THE BIOGRAPHY OF THE CREATOR OF SYNTHETIC INSULIN

EARLY LIFE AND EDUCATION

On November 14th, 1891, Sir Frederick Grant Banting was born to Irish descendants William Thompson Banting and Margret (Grant) Banting, on a small family farm near the small town of Alliston, Ontario just sixty-seven kilometres from Toronto, Ontario (1). The Banting family were active members of the local Methodist Pescatarian Church and had all their children baptized in the local parish (2). Banting, with his blue eyes and light brown hair, was the youngest of five children. He had three brothers, Nelson, William, and Alexander, along with his sister Ester, who was the closest to him in age (2). Growing up on a farm, Banting was used to hard work and being a member of a team of siblings, which might have contributed to his inspiring work ethic and charitable heart. The farm work led Banting to grow up with a robust build and natural athletic abilities, however, his athletic inclination did not follow him into adulthood. (1)

Banting started his journey in education at the local rural school in Alliston, Ontario, which he attended until he completed high school. Banting was noted for having an enquiring mind and a thirst for knowledge (1). Living in a rural part of the country and being the youngest in a family of five children may have negatively impacted Banting's ability to pursue further education. Many children were expected to remain on the property and help with the farm work. However, Banting had a thirst for knowledge that went beyond the fields of his family's farm. His academic drive and natural inclination for learning led to academic success in high school which later resulted in his acceptance into the medical program at Victoria College in the University of Toronto for the fall of 1912 (1). Unfortunately, like many other young men and women, Banting's education was interrupted by the start of World War I.

In the fall of 1915 Banting was one of the many young men that halted their studies to join up with the Canadian Army as part of the Royal Canadian Army Medical Corps (R.C.A.M.C) as an army medic. Banting was originally placed with the Stationary Hospital in Niagara-on-the-Lake from May 4th to October 14th, 1915. It was here that Banting reached the rank of Staff Sergeant Nursing before he was sent home for a few months to complete his medical studies. After graduation, he immediately reenlisted and rejoined as an Officer Lieutenant with the medical corp. Banting was mostly stationed in England but was then moved to France on June 29th, 1918 where he was taken on strength (TOS) with No. 3 Canadian General Hospital. Less than a month later he was TOS on July 14th with the 13th Canadian Field Ambulance before finally being TOSed to the 5th Canadian Field Ambulance on the 18th of August 1918. It was in France that Banting made the rank of Captain while he worked alongside the Field Ambulances assisting in the treatment and transportation of wounded soldiers (2).

Banting has been described as "a most unselfish individual [he] was always mindful of helping others" (3) and it was his selfless nature that led him to receive the Military Cross on December 31st, 1918. The Military Cross is awarded to those who sacrifice their lives in the line of duty to help their fellow countrymen and there is no better reward for Sir Frederick Banting, a war hero and selfless man. Banting Placed himself in the line of fire causing his life to nearly come to an end during the Battle of Cambria on September 28th, 1918. He was wounded via a gunshot wound to his right forearm while doing his duty and providing medical care to wounded soldiers caught in the crossfire (2). Despite the severity of his injury, Banting refused to leave his men untreated. Instead of rushing towards the battalion, and thus to safety, Banting continued to weave through the dropping shells and hailing gunfire to get his men to safety (2). Three days after his injury, Banting was transferred from Ville de Lieges, Belgium to a hospital in Shorncliffe England where he spent the next twenty days fighting for his life. His injury was more severe than originally thought, the bullet had made contact with the bones in his forearm, and there was a period of time where the doctors attending to him believed that the arm might need to be amputated (1). However, after successful surgery, the bullet was removed from his arm and the remaining tissue appeared viable enough to leave intact. Unfortunately, the doctors were not able to reverse the damage the bullet caused to the nerves in his hand and Banting suffered a minor loss of mobility to his little finger (2).

After the war was over, Banting returned to Canada and began his work as a residential surgeon at the Sick Children's Hospital in Toronto (3). He became well known for his skills as an orthopedic surgeon and managed to not be negatively impacted by the loss of mobility in his finger (1). A year later, in 1920, he moved to London, Ontario to start his own practice in medicine. However, his practice was slow to develop leading his inquisitive mind to wander into new projects and he started working as a part-time demonstrator at the University of Western Ontario (2). Working in the medical department at the University of Western Ontario, he began to question the process in which the hormone in the pancreas was being extracted. He believed that the reason previous scientists had been unsuccessful in the extraction was due to the enzymes of the external secretion destroying the internal secretion during the extraction process (2). The idea of his hypothesis being correct was an idea that he was incapable of ignoring. The inquisitive mind and thirst for knowledge and understanding that had been present in his personality since his youth drove him to quit his position at the University of Western Ontario and migrate back to Toronto in search of a research lab where he would be able to test his hypothesis (2). However, finding a willing partner proved to be slightly difficult. Banting had his eye set on John James Rickard Macleod, a well-known professor of physiology at the University of Toronto, who was known internationally in the science community as an expert on carbohydrate metabolism (4). Unfortunately for Banting, Macleod did not consider him a worthy partner as Banting was not an expert in the proposed field and appeared to be unversed in previous experiments that related to Banting's hypotheses. Yet, after speaking with Banting Macleod started to realize the potential for the proposed experiment and the first part of the Insulin discovery team was born (4).

The team grew with the addition of Charles Herbert Best, a recent graduate of the University of Toronto with a B.A Honors in Physiology, who agreed to assist Banting and Macleod in Bantings' dog experiments (4). The aim of the experiment was to first successfully obtain glucose and urine samples from a dog that had a pancreatectomy. Secondly, the team was to go one step further and extract a quantity of pancreatic anti-diabetic solution that was large enough to use in experiments from a fetal calf. After both stages were successfully completed, Banting would inject the dog with the anti-diabetic solution into the dog in an attempt to lower the dog's blood sugar levels. (4)

However, as testing continued Banting became stressed over the morality of animal experimentation. He was aware that the work they were doing was

important to the lives of many people and that in the early stages of experimentation it was simply not safe to conduct human trials. Yet, he was still
troubled by the immoral actions of non-consenting animals being a part of
his experiments and had grown very fond of the dog that was being used in
the trials (1). Therefore, on the 23rd of November, 1921, Banting moved the
experiment from the dog to himself. The first step he took was to inject his
bloodstream with the new extract and once there was no reported adverse
side effect, such as death, he then moved onto step two which was to get
the solution into his digestive system via a feeding tube and wait to see if
there would be any adverse side effects in humans (4). No side effects were
reported, Banting finished the final stage on the dog, which was to have
Best remove an entire dog's pancreas, thus forcing them to become insulin
deficient, and then place the extract into the donor dog's blood to lower the
sugar level in the dog's blood. After the second stage was complete, Banting and the rest of the team felt it was safe to move away from the animal
trials completely and introduce the first human, fourteen-year-old Leonard
Thompson (4).

In 1922 Banting, Macleod, and Best started to receive recognition for their
achievements and the awards started to accumulate. First, in 1922 Banting was the recipient of the Starr Gold Medal for his M.D thesis, which
was then followed by the George Armstrong Peters Prize for the advances
he had facilitated in surgical sciences (1). In 1923 Banting was awarded
both the Reeve Prize and the Charles Mickle fellowship as recognition for
making the most advances in their medical field (1). In 1923, Banting was
also awarded a degree in Doctor of Law from Queen's University while
also completing his Sc.D. from the University of Toronto then again in 1924
from McGill University in Montreal (3). The grand prize and ultimate level
of recognition came in 1923 when both Drs Banting and Macleod were the
recipients of the Nobel Prize in Medicine (1). Bantings' spirit of compassion
and giving is recognizable in the fact that he split the prize money with the
other authors of the work such as Best and Dr. J. B. Collip, a later addition
to the team, while also donating some of his funds to trust to help the young-
er generation reach their potential in both science and art (1).

BANTING: THE ARTIST

The name Sir Frederik Banting and the term 'talented Canadian artist' do
not usually find themselves paced together that often in literature. Yet, art
was one of Banting's greatest pleasures and he was very talented despite the
rocky start of his artistic endeavours. When Banting first decided to start
painting, he walked into an art supply store with little to no knowledge of

the products used by artists. As such, Banting once walked into an art supply store and simply asked for paper and colours, when pressed to explain the types he wanted, he was at a loss of words and just took whatever he could and began experimenting (5). As a self-taught painter, Banting is most famously known for his medical and scientific work, and his artistic skills went unnoticed by many especially in the early years, however, one person that took an interest in Banting's creativity was famous Canadian artist: Alec Jackson who after seeing the work Banting had created, decided to take Banting under his wing and mentor him in post-impressionism and expressionism (5).

Soon the two men became friends and Banting would accompany Jackson to the far northern regions of Canada for inspiration. The trips were physically taxing, and at times they would find themselves beyond the reaches of civilization, yet these trips were artistically stimulating and inspired many of Banting's work (5). Banting was a scientist both in heart and mind and when he started to develop his creative side, he started to see the link between art and science which helped him grow his passion into something more tangible and even considered leaving the scientific practice to become an artist full time by the age of fifty (5). Sadly, Sir Frederik Grant Banting did not live to see his fiftieth birthday.

LEGACY AND LASTING IMPACT

The world came to another halt when German soldiers marched into Poland, thus activating the start of World War II. Historically, the war is remembered as a time of mass destruction and death, and unfortunately, Sir Frederick Grant Banting was not spared as a casualty. When news spread in 1940 that the government was looking to send a medical liaison to work with the British government, Banting was insistent that he should be the one to go (1). Banting never veered from his open-hearted nature, he was a good and kind man that truly dedicated his life to saving others. He was willing to sacrifice himself in the Battle of Cambria, during experimental stages in the pursuit of creating insulin, and again by flying into a country plagued by bombs. On one of his flights to the United Kingdom, Banting's plane crashed in the Newfoundland countryside, he died from his injuries leaving behind a wife and a son; he was forty-nine years old (1).

Banting a man of "courage, persistence, scientific ingenuity and industry" found amusement when his experiments were successful, and it is fair to say that Banting and his team would feel great amusement to know how their discovery of insulin has changed the lives of diabetics for the better (2).

11

Around the time of the invention of artificial insulin, diabetics faced prejudice and were treated as outcasts in society. They did not have equal rights as other citizens, and it even affected their employment opportunities. Dr. John Lister made the claim that they are not fit to work in construction, or in jobs that deal with heavy machinery, which for many blue-collar workers would mean most jobs. P H Sönksen, a member of the Department of Medicine and St Thomas's Hospital Medical School in London, argued that it was wrong and unjustified for medical professionals, such as Dr. John Lister, to claim that diabetics were unfit for scaffolding work. As stated in the article, there were already many legal restrictions placed on diabetics, they were not allowed to obtain a pilot's license, work on or drive on the railway, and it is was not justified to make further claims that they are incapable of holding other forms of employment when there was no evidence that they pose a threat to life. Sönksen points out that Dr. John Lister compared diabetics to alcoholics, who have been proven to cause harm and pose a threat when intoxicated, it is not fair to group someone with underlying health conditions with addicts. Many diabetics are able to hold jobs and work without hypoglycemic reactions, thanks to the invention of insulin and the medical advances discovered by Banting and his team, and should thus be treated with the same respect as non-diabetics (6).

The invention of artificial insulin is one of the greatest scientific discoveries and inventions are known to humankind. Without it, diabetics face shorter lifespans, an increased risk to the development of other health conditions, loss of limbs, comatose state, and even death. Nearly a hundred years after Banting shared his discovery with the world, diabetes is considered to be a manageable condition that allows diabetics to live a healthy and active lifestyle and is no longer seen as an instant death sentence. The impact Banting had on life during his years on Earth is still felt today. He was a war hero, an artist, a father, a doctor, and a scientist, but most importantly he was a creative thinker that refused to quiet the curiosity of the mind.

CHAPTER 3
INSULIN'S IMPACT ON DIABETES

Sameen Ali

Diabetes Mellitus comes from the greek word 'diabetes', meaning to pass through and the latin word 'mellitus' translating to sweet (3). Both these denotations strongly reflect the course of actions that diabetes halts. Diabetes Mellitus is a metabolic disease, indicating that it disrupts the process of food conversion to energy on a cellular level(1, 2). To create energy, our bodies break down food through the digestive system into glucose, a sugar that is then converted to energy through the process of cellular respiration. However, diabetes is the villain that hinders the latter process. To hinder the process, it impacts a crucial organ- the pancreas (9) . This organ is located posterior to the bottom half of the stomach and has the crucial role of making insulin which aids glucose by allowing it to enter cells of our bodies (9, 5). However, diabetes prevents the production of insulin and as a result it is either lacking in quantity or unable to do its assigned task (5). Thus, leading to hyperglycemia which refers to the increased level of blood sugar (4). In this case, the glucose builds up due to the lack of insulin, the deficiency of this important hormone prevents glucose from entering cells and undergoing cellular respiration (2). Hyperglycemia explains the origin of the famous nickname for diabetes - sugar. The chronic hyperglycemia of diabetes also results in long-term damage to organs such as kidneys, nerves, hearts and blood vessels (2). To further understand exactly how insulin impacts diabetes, it is essential to delve into the different types of diabetes and how they influence the essential process. Exactly how does insulin assist glucose in entering cells in a healthy body? What mechanisms do diabetes impede so that it results in complications? What can be done for individuals who have diabetes and how do their bodies cope?

PANCREATIC REGULATION OF GLUCOSE

The human body is dependent on glucose level in the blood in order to maintain normal body function and homeostasis (8). To do this, a network of various hormones and neuropeptides released from the brain, pancreas, liver, intestine and adipose (fat) and muscle tissue is used (8). Amongst these organs and networks, the pancreas plays the key role (8). It regulates digestion hence making it responsible for metabolism by releasing digestive enzymes and pancreatic hormones(8). The pancreas consists mainly of exocrine cells, also known as acinar cells(8). These cells secrete digestive enzymes into the tubes of the pancreas which are known as ducts(8). These ducts have specific names, called accessory pancreatic duct and the main pancreatic duct. The pancreas includes an endocrine function which allows it to release pancreatic hormones directly into the bloodstream(8, 10). The pancreatic islets, which are clusters of cells secrete hormones, one of them being insulin. The pancreas contains five distinct cell types: alpha cells, beta cells, delta cells and PP cells(10). Each type of cell has its own functions and specific hormones that they release. Each hormone has its own function and regulates glucose homeostasis(10).

Mainly through the hormones glucagon and insulin the pancreas maintains blood glucose levels. A normal blood sugar level is less than 7.8mmol/L. A reading of more than 11.1 mmol/L indicates diabetes and a reading of 7.8mmol/L-11mmol/L indicates prediabetes (11). Normal blood sugar is accomplished through glucose homeostasis which refers to glucagon and insulin which are opposing in actions (8). When blood sugar is low, glucagon is released from alpha cells to promote a process called glycogenolysis (8). This process breaks down glycogen - which is the primary carbohydrate stored in the liver - to form glucose. When an individual is fasting for a long period of time, glucagon synthesises oxaloacetate and glycerol in a process called gluconeogenesis (6). An increased rate of gluconeogenesis also contributes to diabetes as it results in more glucose, which increases the blood sugar level (8). In contrast, after eating a meal insulin is secreted from beta cells due to the rising glucose levels. Insulin prevents the blood sugar level from increasing beyond 7.8mmol/L for a nondiabetic patient. However, for a diabetic patient the beta cells are unable to produce insulin leading to the abnormal blood sugar levels (8). After insulin is produced it acts on adipose tissue by enabling the uptake of glucose into these tissues and removing glucose from the bloodstream (8). Insulin is known as an anabolic hormone because it promotes glycogenesis.(8)

Beta cells are signaled to release insulin when the glucose levels in blood sugar are high, this is usually directly after a meal. The glucose is taken up by a facilitative glucose transporter GLUT2, this transporter is located on the surface of beta cells (8). Once the glucose is inside the cell, it undergoes glycolysis - which is the first step in the process of breaking down glucose to extract energy (ATP- adenosine triphosphate), resulting in an increase in ATP/ADP ratio (8). This alteration of ratio signals the closure of ATP-sensitive potassium - channels (K_{ATP}-channels) (8). Under conditions when this channel is not stimulated, the channel is opened allowing K+ ions down their concentration gradient and out of the cell. When the channel is closed, the decrease of K+ -ions outside of the cell results in a depolarization of the membrane which opens the voltage dependent Ca+-channels (VDCC) (8). The increase

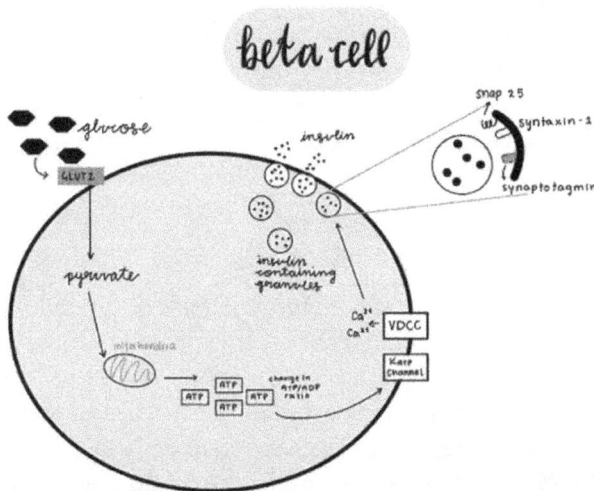

Figure 1. The diagram depicts the secretory pathway of insulin when glucose stimulates the process

in calcium concentration triggers insulin-containing granules that appear as large, dense vesicles to stick to the membrane allowing the vesicle to fuse with the membrane and release the insulin (8). The molecules that aid in the fusion of the vesicle to the membrane creates a SNARE complex, this consists of the proteins, SNAP-25, Syntaxin-1, synaptotagmin (8). Once insulin is secreted into the bloodstream, it travels to the liver, muscle and adipose tissue once it reaches its destination, insulin binds to the insulin receptor attached to the membrane at each location (25). This signals glucose channels and allows glucose to enter the cell through facilitated diffusion (24). However, in patients with diabetes, the body is unable to make enough insulin, locking glucose outside of the cell. In some cases the insulin receptor changes shapes and the insulin is unable to bind to the receptor (42). To explore the details of the process that occurs, let's look at each classification of the disease.

CLASSIFICATION OF DIABETES

There are four main categories of diabetes; however, the vast majority of diabetes cases fall into two main categories: type 1 diabetes, the absolute deficiency of insulin secretion and type 2 diabetes which is a combination of resistance to insulin action and an inadequate insulin secretory response (2). In the latter category, a patient may have hyperglycemia causing functional changes to various target cells; however, without symptoms, it can be present for long periods of time before detection (18). Hyperglycemia can be tissue damaging, in particular it is damaging to cells (2). The other two categories include Gestational diabetes mellitus (GDM) which is diagnosed in the second or third trimester of pregnancy (2). The last category includes specific types of diabetes due to other causes. For example, monogenic diabetes syndromes (such as neonatal diabetes and maturity-onset diabetes of the young (MODY) (2). So, what happens to the regulation of glucose amongst each type of diabetes? Let's discuss this below.

Type 1 Diabetes Type

1 diabetes (T1D) also known as insulin-dependent diabetes or juvenile diabetes is a result of the condition in which the body is unable to make enough insulin to control the blood sugar level (26). Type 1 diabetes is an autoimmune disease, meaning that it begins when the body's immune system attacks cells in the body. In this case, these cells happen to be beta cells — the ones that produce insulin (9, 13). T1D results in the destruction of pancreatic islets, it can occur at any age but is typically common in children at the peak of puberty (16). Genetic factors play a big role in the development of T1D; although there are numerous loci that are involved in the development, only the mechanism of a few are completely known. Having a direct family member such as a sibling or parent can increase the chances of an individual developing diabetes (13). T1D is not caused by the diet an individual has, infact, the disease may be triggered by environmental triggers (13). Similar to the genetic factors, the mechanisms for the majority of the environmental triggers remain unknown. These triggers result in an autoimmune attack of

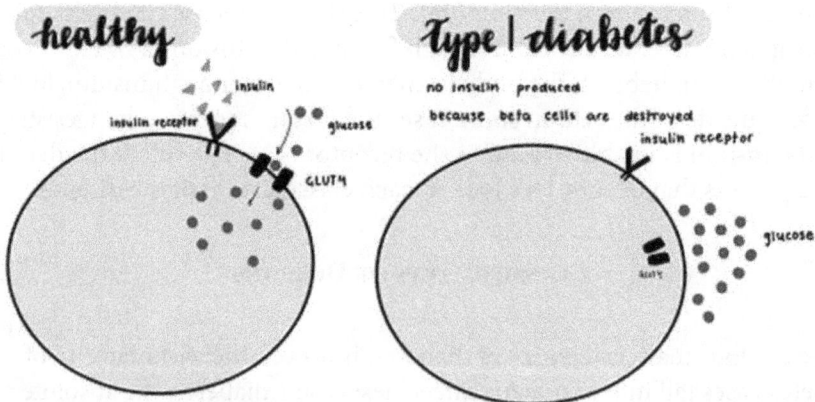

Figure 2. Displays the differences between how a healthy cell uptakes glucose compred to what hinders the diabetic cell with T1D

beta cells in the pancreas that are responsible for carrying out the insulin secretion pathway (13). Without enough beta cells insulin is not produced and as a result insulin receptors are not bound and thus the glucose channels remain closed, locking in glucose into the bloodstream (13).

Although the exact mechanisms for type 1 diabetes is unknown, the genetic region is strongly linked to the human leukocyte antigen (HLA) locus (13). HLA is located on the short arm of chromosome 6 (17). This locus is important to the immune system(11, 13). The strong correlation between genetics and T1D is evident by the fact that 60-65% of identical twins born into a family that has a history of T1D will also develop T1D (12). However, although many twins have the same fate, there is still the remaining percentage that do not. This explains how environmental factors also play a big role. Identical twins may have different fates due to exposure to different environments (13). However, due to the complexity of environmental parameters, their mechanisms of action are mostly unknown. Researchers are looking for a cure to T1D and as a result they have explored new treatments such as islet cell transplant or generating insulin producing cells from stem cells in order to compensate for the dead beta cells (13). However, to truly come up with a solution it is necessary to understand the abnormal changes in the body as a result of this particular type of diabetes (13).

Type 1 diabetes results from the trigger of the immune system against beta cell antigens which stimulates the proinflammatory responses (13). This type of response occurs when cytokines act to make a disease worse (15). Cytokines work in the immune system to respond to infections and any other trauma that may be caused they can respond positively or negatively; however, in this case a negative response is received (15). Antigen-presenting cells (APCs) are immune cells that execute the immune response to an infection; in this case an immunological response occurs because there is inadequate control of the immune response that occured. This leads to beta cell death (13). Beta cell death through an immune response such as this triggers the release of antigens and initiates a similar response to other beta cells, sort of like a domino effect (13).

Some environmental factors that can trigger the development of T1D are obesity and drinking a lot of milk (13). The former is an environmental issue in diabetes that results in increased insulin resistance. The accelerator hypothesis states that obesity-related insulin resistance accelerates the disease process of type 1 diabetes (14). In addition, Children who are overweight have a greater risk of developing T1D. Research has shown that children who consume high amounts of milk products are at a greater risk of autoimmunity against beta cells (13). This is a result of the lack of developing a tolerance to bovine insulin in milk (13). The reaction that bovine insulin triggers in these young children that did not develop a tolerance can cause a critical immune reaction which results in antibodies attacking the human insulin, leading to type 1 diabetes (13).

Type 2 Diabetes

90% of diabetes cases are type 2 diabetes (T2D) . This is most prominent in older people and occurs when the body doesn't produce enough insulin to function properly or if the insulin being produced is not effective (insulin resistance) (27).There is not enough insulin to bind to the receptors or the receptors are unable to bind to insulin at all. This results in the glucose channels remaining closed, increasing blood glucose levels (27). T2D has genetic factors such as age, weight, diet and physical activity. Increased weight increases insulin resistance explaining why obesity plays an important role when it comes to diabetes (27). The main problem arises in the secretion of insulin combined with insulin being unable to bind to its receptors in target tissues such as muscle, liver and adipose tissue (27). In type 2 diabetes, hyperglycemia results when insulin secretion is unable to account for the insulin resistance (27). Insulin is the only hormone in the body that can reduce blood glucose, part of this is due to the fact that having a lower blood sugar is significantly more detrimental than having a higher blood sugar level. If blood sugar falls below 2mmol/L for more than 5 minutes it can be brain damaging (27). Thus the body does not have any other hormone that can perform the same function as insulin.

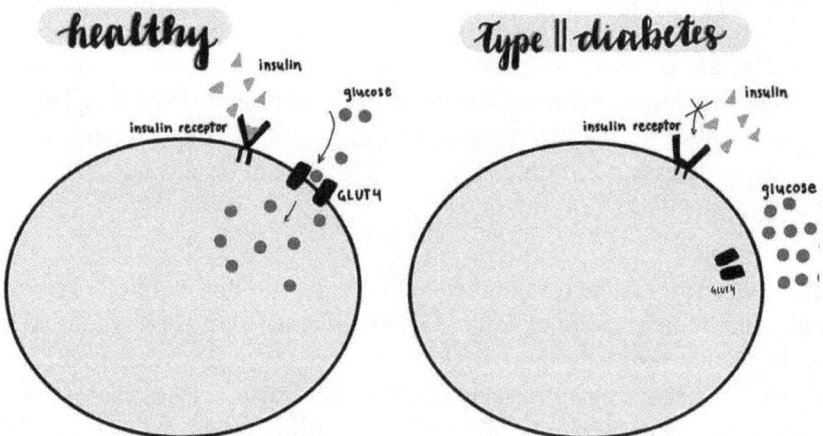

Figure 3. Displays the differences between how a healthy cell uptakes glucose compared to what hinders the diabetic cell with T2D

The lack of insulin in T2D may be due to the lack of secretion of insulin in beta cells. This may be because the beta cell has declined in mass or quantity (27). However, there are various beliefs in exactly why the secretion of insulin is disturbed in type 2 diabetes, a consensus view is lacking. This is partly due to the lack of pancreatic islets present for researching. These islets make up 2% of the human pancreas and play an important role in the secretion of insulin as mentioned before (27). However, the little research that has been conducted on this topic has provided evidence that glucose stimulated insulin secretion is defective in islets from T2D patients relative to non diabetic individuals. This is due to insulin being unable to attach to its receptor to open glucose channels (27). Studies on beta cell mass have been conducted more thoroughly, partly because such studies can be conducted on fixed tissues. Several studies have reported that there is a decrease in beta cell mass in type two diabetes (27). Beta cells can only be detected when there is great insulin concentration available. Thus, beta cells that lack insulin are not seen. Indicating that it has a low mass. A patient who has T2D for 5 years shows a 25% reduction in beta cells that have insulin and long term patients who have had T2D for more than 15 years shows a 50% decrease in insulin-positive cells (27). This significant loss puts greater stress on the cells that do function, and the functionality of these remaining beta cells depends on environmental and genetic factors.

Obesity increases the mass of beta cells by 50% meaning that it does not result in beta cell failure. However, obesity increases T2D because it is primarily associated with insulin resistance (27). Obesity actually enhances insulin response to glucose in non diabetic individuals (27). Aside from weight, another contributing factor to T2D involves changes in beta cells. Changes in beta cell identity may contribute to problems in insulin secretion. This is evident from experimentation done on mice through a situation called beta cell dedifferentiation (27). Mice who have hyperglycemia also have altered expression of beta-cell transcription factors and problems in insulin secretion and recent studies have shown that deletion of certain transcription factors in mice can lead to the dedifferentiation of pancreatic beta cells (27). Dedifferentiation is the reverse process of differentiation, it refers to the loss of special characteristics associated with a cell (19). Thus, in this case when beta cells undergo this situation they lose their insulin concentration and change back into stem cells (27). Although these changes are found in mice, marked changes in beta cell transcription factors have been observed in humans with T2D; however, whether or not the changes in mice exactly reflect those of humans is still unclear (27).

Similar to type 1 diabetes, an individual's risk of developing type two diabetes is determined by both environmental and genetic factors (27). Genotype plays an important role: studies of twins have displayed that out of all the twins that have T2D, 76% of them have the same trait present and 96% of them have impared glucose tolerance (blood sugar is raised beyond the normal level) (27). Similarly, having a family history of T2D doubles the risk of another member obtaining T2D (27). However, many other factors such as lifestyle, food consumption, diet and behaviour have shown evidence of dramatically increasing the rise in T2D over the past 60 years (27).

GESTATIONAL DIABETES MELLITUS (GDM)

Gestational diabetes mellitus (GDM) is a serious illness in which 16.6% of pregnant women worldwide who have never been diagnosed for diabetes develop the condition resulting in high blood glucose level while they are pregnant (22). In most cases this is due to hyperglycemia from pancreatic beta cells dysfunction which is aggravated by insulin resistance (22). Risks increasing the likelihood of obtaining GDM include over weight, high maternal age and having a family history of diabetes. There are also complications that may arise as a result of this disease which includes obtaining T2D, birth complications in the infant, and increased risk of cardiovascular disease (22). GDM can also cause these same complications to arise in the child (22). Similar to T2D and T1D there are management techniques that intervene with insulin; however, a solid cure has not yet been identified.

To understand the pathophysiology of GDM, the regulation of glucose for healthy pregnancies must be viewed. During a healthy pregnancy, the mother's body adapts to the fetus growing within her. Such adaptations include various systems including the metabolic system (22). The most important metabolic adaptation in pregnant women is insulin sensitivity(22). This refers to the effectiveness of insulin binding to the insulin receptor. High insulin sensitivity allows cells to use glucose more effectively, reducing blood sugar (21). Over the course of the pregnancy, insulin sensitivity shifts depending on the requirements. In the earlier stage of pregnancy, insulin sensitivity increases (22). In later stages of the pregnancy hormones such as estrogen, progesterone, leptin, cortisol and placental lactogen promote insulin resistance (22). This causes the blood sugar to elevate since the insulin is unable to bind to its receptors. However, this increased glucose travels to the placenta to fuel the growth of the fetus (22).

Women who have GDM usually do so as a result of beta cell dysfunction and insulin resistance (22). Beta cell dysfunction arises when the secretory pathway of insulin experiences a complication. It is unable to accurately sense glucose and as a result unable to secrete the correct amount of insulin in response. This results in high glucose concentrations (20). The underlying mechanisms that result in beta cell dysfunction can occur at any stage of insulin secretion and synthesis (22). Insulin resistance also just works to increase the issue. The reduced uptake of glucose increases the blood sugar level stressing the beta cells and making them work harder to produce more insulin (22). Insulin resistance also affects GLUT4, the primary glucose transporter. GLUT4 is responsible for bringing glucose into the body and fails to adequately do its assigned task (10, 22). Glucose uptake is reduced by 54% in GDM compared to healthy pregnancies (22).

Conclusion

Insulin is a crucial hormone; a suitable nickname may be "the goldilock hormone" since too much is deadly but too little is also detrimental. It plays an important role in glucose regulation and in the many cases that it fails to adequately perform its job, the outcome is diabetes. Diabetes is a disease that is so incredibly widespread yet complicated due to all the mechanisms involved in the process. Although researchers have found a great deal of information on the disease, a lot more is still left to unravel and discover. Researchers have managed to use the knowledge so far to find methods to control each type of diabetes. However, they have yet to obtain the information that will aid in finding the cure for not one but all types of diabetes. Perhaps with more progress in technology and resources available all the underlying causes of diabetes can be tackled and a long term solid cure can be provided depending on the type of diabetes an individual has been diagnosed with. Insulin has a great impact on diabetes and must be focused on for this critical research

Chapter 4
What is Insulin?

Belinda Tam
For the Antarctic Institute of Canada
May 8, 2021

The very definition of insulin can come in many different ways depending on the context in which the word is being used. When individuals first think about insulin, what comes to mind is a drug used to treat diabetic patients. However, it is also a hormone that is secreted by the human body.

In terms of anatomy, insulin is defined as a peptide hormone secreted by beta (β) cells in the pancreas. Insulin has many functions including regulating blood sugar levels in the human body, regulating carbohydrate, lipid, and protein metabolism, promoting cell division, and growth. When the pancreas does not produce enough insulin, it causes diabetes. (For more information on diabetes, please refer to the chapter before.) For a healthy human being, the pancreas secretes insulin into the bloodstream. As insulin spreads throughout the body, chemical reactions occur in cells which result in blood sugar entering blood cells. When the blood sugar reaches an appropriate level in the body, the pancreas stops producing insulin. With that being said, blood sugar plays a vital role in this process as it provides the body with energy for building muscles, tissue, and brain. Without blood sugar, doing those key activities would be very difficult and larger problems may occur including "nerve damage, kidney damage, blindness, skin conditions, and hearing impairment".(3)

Individuals who have diabetes are often given periodic insulin injections to regulate their blood sugar to minimize the symptoms associated with diabetes (generally). What is interesting about this is that although the injections are painful for patients, researchers hypothesize that the pain felt with administering insulin may actually come from the size and sharpness of the needle and/or how much insulin is injected.(4) The researchers test this theory with diabetic patients and end up concluding that the level of pain is associated with how hard the needles are injected, not by the size or volume of the needle and injection. In saying that, this is an area of future research that can be further developed to see if different types of needles might be better suited towards different situations as currently, hospitals use syringe-needles while those doing it by themselves use preloaded insulin pens.

STRUCTURE AND CHEMICAL PROPERTIES OF INSULIN

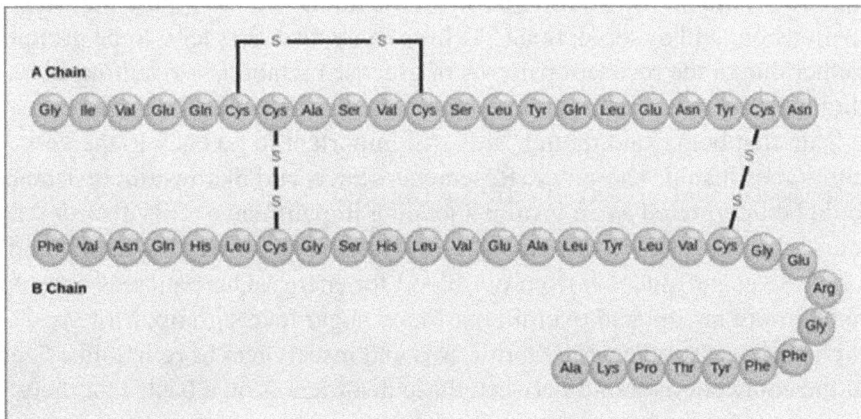

Figure 1

Insulin was originally found to be a single polypeptide protein, meaning that it is a single line of multiple amino acids, while it was later identified as a dipeptide containing A and B chains respectively, being linked by disulfide bridges and containing 51 amino acids. In reference to the image above, A chain contains 21 amino acids while chain B has 30 amino acids. The S on the figure represents the disulfide bridges.(8)

CHEMICAL REACTIONS

As insulin causes a variety of chemical reactions it is important to define some of the key reactions if we are to define the word insulin. Firstly, insulin can trigger a variety of metabolic reactions. Depending on which metabolic pathways are impacted by this hormone, insulin can be defined differently. Some examples of this include lipid and protein metabolism and the processes associated with them – lipogenesis and protein synthesis.(5) Lipogenesis is a process involving fatty acid and triglyceride synthesis being controlled and regulated by numerous factors in the body. The process is stimulated by a diet concentrated in carbohydrates and hormones in the body, including insulin.(4)

Moreover, insulin resistance has become a major type of chemical reaction as altered patterns of glucose metabolism and a variety of disorders are associated with it. Having insulin resistance can also lead to heart attacks, stroke, and kidney disease. One of the major disorders that are associated with insulin resistance is the insulin resistance syndrome. This syndrome includes a variety of problems including obesity, high blood pressure, and type 2 diabetes.(5) Currently, research associated with this area has been used to help understand the connection between disorders such as type 2 diabetes, hypertension, and dyslipidemia.(5) These three disorders tend to be grouped together due to the resistant patterns of glucose metabolism resulting in individuals often associating these disorders with upper abdominal excess fat. With that being said though, it is still important to go back to the very definition of insulin resistance. Researchers have said that insulin resistance should be interpreted as an insulin signaling impairment as this disorder occurs when the cells in our muscles no longer respond well to insulin and cannot use sugar(glucose) from our blood for energy. Our pancreas ends up making more insulin and overall, our blood sugar levels go up. More research still needs to be done on this area and researchers have hypothesized that the connections found between these disorders is on a basis that there are more than one phenotype playing a key role in these illnesses in our modern society. Further research may also look into how insulin may affect individuals differently depending on their body composition as there are no common traits for insulin resistance and factors that are listed are purely environment based "or acquired factors that cause or aggravate insulin resistance."(5)

MEDICINE & INNOVATION

According to Baeres et al., innovation is "a new method, idea, or product." (1) The researchers who wrote this article believe that developing better therapies through incremental improvement of existing products is a form of innovation. This concept is explored in this article through an insulin analogue development to better innovate products for individuals with diabetes.

In this regard, it is essential to discuss the types of insulin and insulin analogues. Firstly, there are five types of insulin analogues – rapid acting, short acting, intermediate acting, long acting, and mixtures. Rapid acting insulin works over a short range of time and is usually used at the beginning of a meal. If used at the start of dinner, it may prevent severe drops in

24

blood sugar levels in the middle of the night. Out of the five types of insulin analogues, they are most similar to the type produced by the pancreas since it quickly drops the blood sugar level for a short duration. In comparison, short acting insulin are most often used 30 to 60 minutes before a meal so it has time to work in the body. Intermediate and long acting insulin contain substances to make them work over a long period of time. Lastly, mixtures of insulin is an interesting category as some types of insulin can be combined whereas others cannot and the functions of certain combinations have not been figured out yet so this may be a very interesting area of research to go into. With that being said, a variety of insulins fall into these five types of analogues. Please find a table below that includes some examples of insulin that fall into each type of analogue. (9)

Type	Example	When it Starts to Work (Onset Time)	How Long does it last (Duration)
Rapid Acting	Fiasp (faster-acting insulin aspart)	4 Minutes	3.5 - 5 Hours
Short Acting	Entuzity (insulin regular)	15 minutes	17 – 24 hoursw
Intermediate acting	Humulin N, Novolin ge NPH	5-8 hours	Up to 18 hours
Long acting	Tresiba (degludec)	1.5 hours	42 hours

Table 1

These types of analogues and insulins have been integrated into products by companies who were using various protein engineering techniques so that the product created would be better suited for individuals and their needs. That said, although creating a new product will require testing, there may still be the possibility that the created product will not work for every single customer. The company can only do its best with the information that they have and that is coming in from the field (i.e. pharmacotherapy). Specifically, for those who have diabetes, purchasing a product may in turn help with better meeting their various needs, "resulting in individuals being able to manage [the condition]."(1) On a larger scale, this will hopefully positively impact individuals when using the product well "and provide an opportunity for owners to significantly improve their everyday lives." (1) When comparing the analogue regimen discussed in the Baenes article to other insulin analogues, it was found that the technique is advantageous from both the safety and efficacy viewpoint. This demonstrates the high potential that incremental refinement of one drug can have to the field. At the end of this article, both the researchers and readers are well informed that making small changes to existing therapies can be just as impactful to the field as completely new therapies.

In relation back to this chapter – what is insulin, we find another way to define this word. Depending on the area that it is integrated with, in this case merging healthcare with innovation, what results depends on how the concept is applied. For future research, seeing how insulin can impact other beings such as plants or further research being done on other mammals could be beneficial to not only healthcare but other fields as well.

Insulin, Obesity, and Pregnancy

Although these three topics may seemingly be uncorrelated, in this section I will discuss how they are related with a large focus put on obesity. Normal pregnancy is characterized by insulin resistance, with the greatest amount during the third trimester. This seems to be a response to diverting glucose and lipids into the developing fetus. In relation to obesity, this may be why we see women gaining more weight on the upper body. Generally, increased adipose tissue in the upper body was first associated with diabetes in vascular disease by Jean Vague in 1956. Although this obviously differs between individuals, "weight gain worsens and weight loss improves insulin resistance in those who are predisposed" (11). Especially for women who are obese, "they are at increased risk for having decreased insulin sensitivity [in] comparison with lean or average weight women. This combination of obesity and decreased insulin sensitivity increases the long term risk of these individuals developing the metabolic syndrome and associated problems of diabetes, hypertension, hyperlipidemia and cardiovascular disorders." (3) In relation to pregnancy, women who are obese will likely have decreased insulin sensitivity and are at increased risk for various pregnancy outcomes." (3)

Body Composition of the Fetus

When this topic was originally researched, the assessment of how the fetus grew has been categorized and described in various ways. In the later part of the last century, we have been categorizing people growth according to birth weight as a function of gestational age. Further descriptions of the estimation of body composition include lean and fat mass percentage with the average fat mass being 10 to 12% approximately. For lean body mass, it has been said that it has a stronger correlation with genetic factors in comparison to mass as it may relate more to the maternal environment.(3) However, it is important to use body composition when assessing fetal growth in relation to the utero environment.

Relating this back to obese women though, researchers have identified that infants birthed from obese woman "weigh more at birth than either women with weight matched normal glucose tolerance or normal weight women, respectively." (3) One may ask why this is the case so further research has been done on this and researchers have learned that infants birthed from obese woman weigh more because the mother gains more fat mass and not lean body mass. A strong correlation has also been found between neonatal fat mass in women with Gestational Diabetes Mellitus (GDM) and decreased maternal pregravid (preceding pregnancy) insulin sensitivity. "In obese women, maternal pregravid BMI, as a surrogate for insulin resistance, has the strongest correlation with neonatal adiposity. The increased adiposity at birth is also a risk factor for childhood obesity and long term metabolic dysfunction." (3)

In reference to the health and innovation section of this chapter, insulin analogues can be used in relation to pregnancy as well. According to Lambert et al, having a strong glycaemic control is vital during pregnancy to have maternal and fetal outcomes. In the paper, they "aim to assess the efficacy and safety of insulin analogues in pregnancy [using insulin lispro and insulin aspart as examples]." (6) It is noted that "insulin analogues may offer potential benefits over human insulin and many pregnant women with type 1 diabetes are using insulin analogues at conception." (10) Although much research is still to be done on this area before insulin analogues can be recommended to pregnant women universally.

To summarize, maternal obesity and insulin resistance are major short and long term risk factors for the mother and her fetus. For obese women with decreased insulin sensitivity, pregnancy poses as a stress test for disorders

associated with pregnancy and whether or not these disorders are going to be carried with them long term for both the mother and her child.

In saying that, the offspring are at a higher risk of disorders such as neonatal morbidity and childhood metabolic dysfunction. Childhood metabolic dysfunction may cause a vicious cycle of obesity and insulin resistance for the generations that follow. Therefore, having a healthy diet, maintaining exercise, and weight control before and during gestation offers the possibility of short and long term benefit for both the mother and her child. To conclude, why care what insulin is? One major reason would be that there is currently no cure for diabetes and unfortunately, this disorder is becoming more and more common in our society everyday. Insulin as a whole then, can be described as a mitigator, a solution, to help individuals control this better in their everyday lives. As this chapter shows, there are many definitions of the word insulin – how it is being described in anatomy, how it is connected to chemical reactions, innovation, to obesity, pregnancy, and body composition, this term can mean a variety of things. I have described a few definitions of the word insulin in this chapter but there are many other ways to define the word insulin. Future researchers can focus on how this word can be utilized in other areas such as engineering.

CHAPTER 5
BARRIERS TO ACCESS: ESSENTIAL INSULIN FOR DIABETES

Avery Kennedy
For the Antarctic Institute of Canada
May 6th 2021

Many factors can act as barriers at every stage of diagnoses and treatment of diabetes. Factors such as lack of resources, race, and insulin non-adherence can all contribute to a patient's inability or unwillingness to use insulin therapy. These barriers can also affect the quality of care patients receive and can lead to years of delay in appropriate, sometimes necessary, commencement and adjustment of insulin treatment.

Lack of resources is a significant barrier to access to insulin and diabetes treatment. A study done in rural, underprivileged populations in South Texas found evidence that, "Health disparities are often geographically bound and occur more frequently in impoverished populations."[2] This makes sense as rural areas often have less access to technology and specialists, and underprivileged people in these areas have less of an ability to pay for such treatments. In a country like the United States, where diabetes is the seventh leading cause of death, [6] insulin and healthcare in general is incredibly expensive. Therefore, people without the means to do so, struggle to get the treatment they need, especially in rural and underprivileged areas. "Studies have shown that rural youth with type 1 diabetes even globally has higher rates of hospital admissions, lower appointment adherences and poorer communication with their care team." compared to their counterparts in cities.[5]

 The situation is actually worse than it may seem because diabetes can lead to many further complications. Lack of resources is a principle cause of conditions related to diabetes such as retinopathy.[5] Of course, there are ways to ameliorate the situation. In a study done in rural India, they concluded that the use of insulin pumps would likely have an overwhelmingly positive effect on the quality of life of rural, underprivileged patients with type 1 diabetes. They recommend studies on the use of a technology called Carelink, which is an electronically based system to monitor and adjust insulin levels. It would reduce the need for hospital visits. However, all of these technologies are very expensive and would require the assistance of government, NGOs and the industry to become accessible for those with socioeconomic barriers.[5]

Race also plays a part in access to healthcare and insulin. A study done in the United States on a Hispanic population with type two diabetes found "Adult Hispanics continue to have more unmet health care needs compared to non-Hispanic Whites because of cost factors. In particular, the lack of insurance."[3] States choosing not to expand Medicaid also has an adverse effect in Hispanic populations. A lack of culturally competent health care providers was also an issue the study highlighted. The study suggested that physicians who can work outside of typical business hours, who offer service in Spanish, and who have an understanding of the patient's' culture, especially as it relates to family support and stigma in the community, would have a huge impact on the accessibility of care in the community and would help insulin non-adherent patients get the treatment they need.[3]

Insulin non-adherence is an umbrella term that covers many factors. One study categorizes these factors as self, provider, and environment barriers that deter patients from proper insulin treatment. Self-barriers are factors that come from your life experience, though are not necessarily in your control. Age, education, and stigma originating from culture are all self-barriers. The study also includes a subcategory of individual resources, which includes the expenses involved with insulin therapy as well as diabetic friendly foods, expenses related to fitness, and the time, consuming process of seeking and keeping up with treatment. [3]

A literature review of studies on barriers to insulin in cases with type 2 diabetes found that insulin non-adherent patients were more worried about their ability to adjust insulin dosage, side effects like hypoglycemia, and insulin's potential impact on their quality of life. There were also many with injection anxiety. Some did not adhere because they planned on changing their lifestyle or because they felt insulin was not necessary. There was a common belief that insulin was a punishment of sorts for not taking care of themselves and many blamed themselves for their condition. [4]

Healthcare provider barriers are categorized as an unavailability of healthcare providers and a lack of communication between healthcare providers and patients. Distance to treatment, lack of trust and long waitlists were also barriers to providers. In the same literature review, they found that patients who were non-adherent received less or no insulin self-management training from their health care provider compared to the insulin adherent. Many felt their healthcare provider "failed to adequately explain insulin's risk and benefits"[4] and "35% of the insulin-non adherent group reported that they believed insulin causes harm" such as blindness, amputations, heart attacks, and early death. They also reported not understanding the written information they had access to about their condition.[4] The review concluded that addressing the lack of communication and proper education between healthcare providers and patients will likely help absolve these barriers and lead more patients who are inexperienced with insulin to adhere to their prescriptions.

Finally, environmental barriers were defined as a lack of information or services and any language barriers between patients and healthcare providers or information.[3] This applies especially in the study's context of the Hispanic communities in the United States but as demonstrated by the literature review referenced above, is applicable even when there is no language barrier present. The level of education on insulin had a crucial impact on people's beliefs about insulin and their view of themselves and their condition. The environment also plays a part in your physical access to healthcare. As previously discussed, people living in rural areas or without close access to a hospital will see less treatment, even without factoring in their access to specialists such as opticians, dentists, and nutritionists who are vital in raising the quality of life of patients with diabetes and ensuring they are being treated appropriately for their condition.[6]

Diabetes education can play a critical role in the well-being of diabetic patients. The term non-adhering is placing all the blame on the patient when it is in fact a culmination of variables often including patient education and healthcare practitioner communication. The role of specialists and healthcare practitioners is vital for teaching patients about the treatments they are being prescribed, comprehensive meal plans which aim to improve the overall health of patients, and an understanding of the importance that lifestyle plays in diabetes management are vital resources for patients with diabetes. Different specialists and effective communication with healthcare practitioners can aid in setting goals and ensuring an understanding of the goals so the patients are incentivised to stick with them.[6]

Another study focusing on the lack of treatment patients who had access to insulin were receiving also highlighted several barriers in different stages of treatment. These patients' blood glucose level targets were not met for years before their insulin levels were increased; especially in patients with little knowledge of insulin.[1] The study identified three main causes at the clinical and patient level initiation, titration, and intensification inertia. They described initiation inertia as a delayed initiation of insulin, titration inertia as a lack of dose adjustment, and intensification inertia as delayed intensification of dosage.

Studies done in the UK overtime show that the time between reaching above target levels of glucose and progressing from oral antidiabetic treatments to insulin can be anywhere from two to eight years. Multinational studies have shown that the rates vary between countries but this inertia appears globally. The consequence of this initiation inertia is that patients are not receiving the appropriate care they need at the appropriate time. This can lead to any of the side effects associated with untreated diabetes. The reasons for this initial lack of care vary from the risk of hypoglycemia to difficulty following a regimen. Around 30% of people with diabetes they polled found following a schedule to be difficult. Hesitancy also stemmed from the perceived possibility of weight gain, fears surrounding injection, self-measuring blood glucose, and change of lifestyle, as well as a perception of failure in the case of type 2 diabetics. Some of them saw insulin treatment as a punishment for failing to make lifestyle changes rather than the lifesaving treatment it can offer. The study suggested that another important factor could be lack of experience by healthcare professionals in initiating insulin, especially in the case of primary care physicians as opposed to specialists. Simply by virtue of their job, primary care specialists are likely to have less time to address issues surrounding insulin and a lack of access to specialists can make it very difficult to receive the care the patients need.

One of the solutions the study proposes is the initiation of insulin being led by nurse practitioners. According to the study, they are in a better position to administer and address issues or concerns because of more frequent contact with the patients during their ongoing use of insulin. General practitioners have less contact with patients and typically address multiple issues in a single appointment, and there is evidence that the involvement and education of nurse practitioners leads to a more accurate intensification of treatment. Another solution they propose is improving long-acting analogue devices. They can provide a more consistent delivery of insulin and lower risk of hypoglycemia, which could reduce patient hesitancy surrounding insulin treatment. The third and vital solution is education and communication between the different healthcare practitioners treating a patient and said patient. They are in an important position to address concerns the patient may have and to alleviate patient concerns about drastic and burdensome lifestyle changes. They can also reduce fear and lack of education as a barrier for the insulin naive. The study recommends a psychologist with knowledge of diabetes be available to help patients with severe psychological barriers to initiation. They also discuss the importance of a psychologist in the case of a patient with depression or anxiety, which have been shown to have a negative impact on initiation as well as compliance.[1]

With titration inertia, many of the issues with initiation carry over to dose adjustment. A lack of healthcare professional resources to attend to patients can mean delays in dose adjustment. Patient fear about hypoglycemia and weight gain can also play a part in delaying increases in insulin dosage. This, among other factors, can lead patients to omit insulin or not check their blood glucose levels frequently enough due to a fear of major lifestyle changes. The study highlights that healthcare practitioners can contribute to these issues through lack of communication and failure to emphasise the importance of these treatments and alleviate the patient's fear. They reference some real world studies that show factors that can contribute to the probability of adherence or non-adherence. Factors increasing non-adherence probability include being a student, a prescription with lots of injections, and having a type 2 diabetes diagnosis as opposed to a type 1 diagnosis. Factors increasing adherence probability include "support from a diabetes nurse specialist, (...) hypoglycemia awareness, following a healthy diet, perceived self efficacy and previous experience of liaison psychiatry or cognitive behavioral therapy."[1]

The study proposes some solutions including less complicated regimens that are patient-led and diabetes self-management education that helps manage treatment and develop good habits. There have been some mixed results in long-term studies but there are absolutely short-term improvements. Other possible solutions include new devices and applications to help manage dosage, track food intake and require less contact with physicians. Mobile apps especially have some promising results but do need more development. It is important to keep in mind that apps and technology have promising, albeit varied, results in studies where apps were used by elderly patients and the study concludes that more studies should be done to get conclusive and long-term data on some of these areas.

Intensification inertia is the delayed intensification of dosage overtime, which is sometimes needed in patients with type 2 diabetes. The intensification comes in many forms, which include adding a bolus insulin or the addition of non-insulin agents for the prevention of hypoglycemia. There are similar contributing factors to intensification inertia as the previous types such as injection anxiety in patients, more complex routines, the risk or fear of adverse side effects, and lack of time on the part of the physician to make an appropriate diagnosis. One suggested solution was the use of a new medication that is combined with insulin in a once per day shot. This would help keep routines uncomplicated therefore limiting the lifestyle impact and lowering patient non-adherence. In several studies done globally, they have found that healthcare providers agree to varying degrees that the system would benefit from "specialist nurse availability, psychological support, and earlier diagnosis and treatment." [1] These changes would increase communication between patients and healthcare providers, help ameliorate patient education, and ensure that more time could be spent on each patient making their condition easier to diagnose and manage for the healthcare providers.

CHAPTER 6
SCIENTIFIC EVIDENCE SUPPORTING INSULIN THERAPY

John Christy Johnson

INTRODUCTION

In this chapter, we will consider the primary goals of standard insulin therapy and briefly touch on some of the specialized scenarios in which insulin treatment is indicated. We will talk about glycemic control and the different types of ways in which we can regimen insulin to achieve patient glycemic targets. Afterwards, an exposition of these glycemic targets will be explored as they relate to Type 1 (T1DM) and Type 2 (T2DM) Diabetes Mellitus. T1DM and T2DM both have some common medical emergencies associated with them (diabetic ketoacidosis and hyperglycemic hyperosmolar syndrome) in which insulin therapy serves as a mainstay treatment.

Subsequently, there will be a few sections dedicated towards other uses of insulin therapy including complications in pregnancy, endocrine human growth hormone disorders, and its use in performance enhancement. Finally, we discuss and conclude with some of the need-to-know risks of insulin therapy.

GLYCEMIC CONTROL AND INSULIN THERAPY

Glycemic control is well-recognized as a major factor preventing the complications of diabetes in both patients with T1DM and T2DM. Hyperglycemia is a major risk factor for not only microvascular complications such as retinopathy, nephropathy, and neuropathy but also macrovascular complications such as heart attacks.

The American Diabetes Association generally recommends a hemoglobin A1C level of less than 7% although targets are often modified to suit outpatient goals and outcomes.

TYPES OF THERAPIES

A series of complex insulin regimens are employed to achieve desired effects in diabetic patients. To simplify, the major regimens include short-acting, higher-effect bolus insulin; longer-acting, lower-effect basal insulin; and/or some mixture of these. Similarly, there are also different routes of administration for insulin including by syringe, by pen, and by pump.

While the lexicon for diabetes therapies is elusively varied, three major forms of insulin therapies can be parsed out in order of use:

1) Augmentation therapy: the use of basal and bolus insulin as an adjunct to residual β-cell insulin
2) Replacement therapy: the use of basal and bolus insulin as a substitute for endogenous β-cell insulin
3) Rescue therapy: the use of bolus insulin as an acute (scale of weeks) therapy to mitigate dangerously high levels of blood glucose

Of these, augmentation therapy is the most common and typically used in T2DM, where the hallmark is progressive loss of pancreatic β-cells. Randomized clinical trials have shown strong effects of basal insulin in lowering fasting blood glucose and of bolus insulin in lowering postprandial (or postmeal) blood glucose levels.

Replacement therapy is commonly used in T1DM and T2DM patients who have completely lost insulin function. The use of replacement therapy has been associated with a 11% reduction in 3-year mortality for patients who have experienced a heart attack, 46% reduction in sepsis, 42% reduction in dialysis, and 50% reduction in transfusions.

Note that rescue therapy is typically reserved for diabetic emergencies including acute illness, post-surgery complications, pregnancy, diabetic ketoacidosis, and glucose toxicity. In some cases, it has been shown that acute interventions of insulin rescue therapy can actually preserve insulin function for months or years.

There is also evidence to suggest that using metformin (T2DM antihyper-glycemic agent) in conjunction with insulin is associated with better health outcomes including reduced incidences of hypoglycemia and less weight gain. It is also cost-effective when compared to traditional triple oral medi-cation (sulfonylureas, metformin, thiazolidinediones) with a cost saving of over $7/day. This can not only save enough for a blood glucose monitor for those who are socioeconomically disadvantaged, but also allow the patient to obtain the same HbA1C-lowering effect as someone on a triple oral med-ication. [1]

T1DM Evidence

The Diabetes Control and Complications Trial (DCCT) and the Epidemi-ology of Diabetes Interventions and Complications (EDIC) are landmark studies that demonstrated intensive glycemic control can significantly reduce chronic complications in T1DM [2]. The study split off cohorts into a con-trol conventional therapy group and another that used three or more daily insulin injections or self-monitored insulin pump therapy to bring HbA1C levels to normal range.

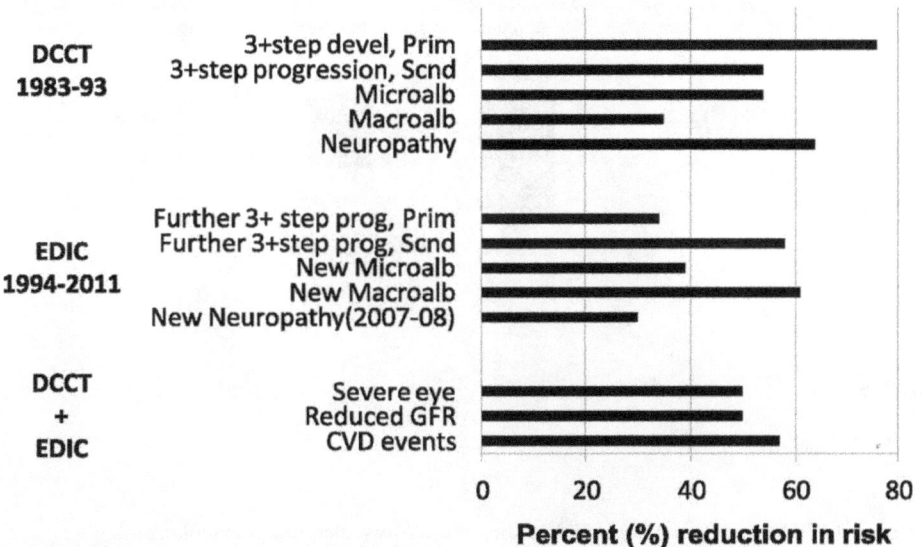

Figure 1: DCCT and EDIC reductions in T1DM patients' microvascular, macrovascular, and other complications with intensive glycemic control. [2] The EDIC was a follow-up of members from the DCCT cohort and as such, built off the previous complications [2] .

As shown in the figure, several major diabetic complications including retinopathy complications (indicated by the 3+step devel, Prim and 3+step progression, Scnd in DCCT and indicated by the Further 3+step prog, Prim and Further 3_step prog, Scnd in EDIC). Microalbuminuria and subsequent macroalbuminuria are other complications that were reduced. Additionally, neuropathy, which often presents as diabetic foot, was also noted to be reduced. In both studies, it was noted that eye symptoms were not as severe as the conventional therapy group. Furthermore, the glomerular filtration rate (GFR), an indicator of kidney function, showed much better values in comparison to the conventional therapy group. This also suggests the reduced risk of nephropathy or kidney complications, yet another type of microvascular complication.

T2DM Evidence

The United Kingdom Prospective Diabetes Study (UKPDS) was a key study that demonstrated intensive glycemic control can significantly reduce chronic complications in T2DM. A caveat for this study was that sulfonylureas (one of the triple oral antihyperglycemic medications) was also used for the purposes of HbA1C lowering. Regardless, the point is that glycemic control, whether it be by insulin or any other agent, is beneficial.

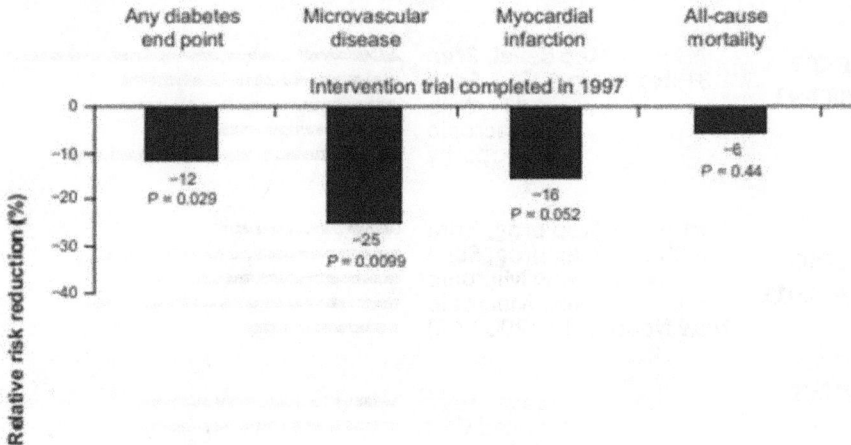

Figure 2: UKPDS reductions in T2DM patients' microvascular, macrovascular, and other complications with intensive glycemic control. [3]

The study, quite similar to DDCT and EDIC, was able to show how glycemic control, an 11% lower HbA1c showed significantly better outcomes with regard to microvascular complications like nephropathy, neuropathy, and retinopathy and macroscopic complications like heart attacks over the first 10 years. There was also an overall reduction in the progression of the disease (Any disease end point) and a lowering of all-cause mortality, meaning that subjects in the treatment group generally lived longer.

DIABETIC KETOACIDOSIS

Diabetic ketoacidosis is a medical emergency, typically seen in T1DM, characterized by high blood glucose, blood ketones, dehydration, and metabolic acidosis. What compounds this situation is that the body has inadequate reserves of insulin for its metabolic processes. Oftentimes, diabetic patients presenting with diabetic ketoacidosis may have accidentally forgotten to have taken their insulin or may have infection or another illness that precipitated this state. In this scenario, although the first line of treatment is fluid therapy, insulin is also used to turn off ketones and glucose production.

In pediatric diabetes patients, another complication associated with diabetic ketoacidosis is cerebral edema causing or caused by the swelling of certain neurons. This is crucial to correct to prevent long-term damage to the child's brain development and a high-risk sequelae of decompensatory pathophysiology. Additionally, because most children with new onset diabetes have T1DM, they are at an even higher risk of progressing to cerebral edema in diabetic ketoacidosis.

Insulin also deals with another physiological repercussion in this state. During acidotic states, potassium ions start leaking out of cells. This is a result of the body's compensatory mechanism to shift the acid from the blood into cells. Insulin can actually cause the potassium ions to be returned to the cells thereby preventing a hyperkalemic (high potassium ion) state. Normally, we do not have to worry about hyperkalemia but in the case of a diabetic ketoacidosis patient, there is a need to replenish potassium ions intravenously that is lost from dehydration.

HYPERGLYCEMIC HYPEROSMOLAR SYNDROME

Hyperglycemic Hyperosmolar Syndrome is another medical emergency, typically seen in T2DM, characterized by a relative insulin deficiency, impaired glucose uptake, and more glucose production by the liver. The result is an excessive amount of glucose in the blood that starts disrupting the osmotic gradient of water between the intracellular and extracellular environments. The most concerning symptom appears when the hyperosmolarity starts affecting brain cells and drawing water out causing impairments in consciousness. In most cases, there are intercurrent illnesses, infections or other medications involved. In these types of instances, once again insulin is a crucial part of the treatment approach. Cautious administration of insulin can effectively reverse the hyperglycemic hyperosmolar state.

GESTATIONAL DIABETES MELLITUS & PREGNANCY

For diabetic mothers in early pregnancy or who are planning a pregnancy, replacement therapy insulin is recommended. Major congenital anomalies including impaired brain size, musculoskeletal defects, and urogenital complications were reduced in those mothers who were treated to match standard glycemic targets during pregnancy. [4]

During late pregnancy, even the normoglycemic mother is at an increased risk of acquiring higher blood glucose states. Currently, there are several uncontrolled studies that suggest an association between hyperglycemia and negative outcomes for the fetus and the mother. One problem that arises is dystocia, or obstructed labour. While the first line of treatment is typically dietary, rescue therapy insulin will have to be used in more serious blood glucose lowering interventions. [5]

MALIGNANT HYPERTHERMIA

Malignant hyperthermia is a hypermetabolic disorder that can arise from potent inhalation agents (halothane, sevoflurane, desflurane and succinylcholine) and in rarer instances, heavy exercise and intense heat. These inhalation agents are typically used in anesthetic procedures and as such, is a common hospital-induced condition. Some of the hallmark signs of this syndrome include increased heart rate, respiration rate, increased CO_2 production, increased O_2 consumption, acidosis, muscle rigidity, and rhabdomyolysis. As a result, the body starts depleting its ATP sources, the muscle membranes start becoming structurally compromised. This can lead to potassium ion leakage and hyperkalemia.

As aforementioned in the diabetic ketoacidosis section, insulin can actually cause the potassium ions to be returned to the cells thereby preventing a hyperkalemic state. Oftentimes, the acidemia and hyperkalemia can be jointly treated using a combination of hyperventilation, bicarbonate, glucose/insulin, and calcium. The insulin coupled with the glucose ensures effective blood glucose uptake.

It may be important to note that insulin is a mitogenic compound. This means that insulin akin to steroids can be used as a mediator of cellular and tissue-level growth. In excess quantities, it can also mediate disadvantageous cancerous-like growth and hyperproliferation of cells particularly in the context of insulin resistance and diabetes.

In insulin resistance states, high insulin levels can stimulate IGF-1 production in the liver. This becomes important in the treatment of syndromes of growth hormone insensitivity. As shown below, IGF-1 has a plethora of effects on metabolism in the body that affect parts of the reproductive, immune, musculoskeletal, and cardiovascular system. [6]

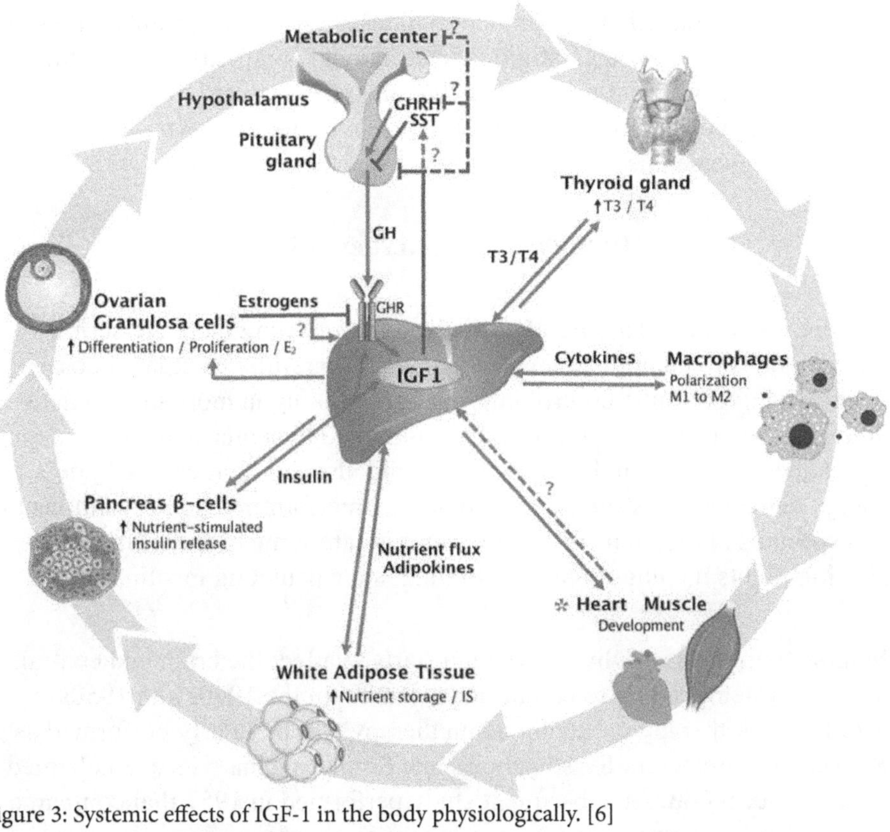

Figure 3: Systemic effects of IGF-1 in the body physiologically. [6]

It is also worth noting that IGF-1 and insulin receptors have a common homology. And while the growth hormone-IGF-1 axis primarily controls tissue growth and differentiation and insulin cascade primarily controls fuel metabolism, these systems can cross-talk. While mechanistically unclear, the scientific literature suggests that IGF-1 analogue therapy and combination therapy with insulin produce positive effects on both T1DM and T2DM states of insulin resistance. [7]

INSULIN AS A PERFORMANCE-ENHANCING DRUG

Bodybuilders have been trying to capitalize on the anabolic effects of insulin to promote performance and enhance stamina. Similar to testosterone and human growth hormone, insulin can consolidate muscle tissue. Unfortunately, excessives of this practice is one that is not to be recommended and on the contrary, can be quite dangerous. Overdosing on insulin can induce the dangerous cerebral symptoms of hypoglycemia.

In 1998, a non-diabetic German bodybuilder attempted to stimulate muscle growth directly before a prestigious international competition. Unfortunately, the short acting insulin he took subcutaneously resulted in a hypoglycemic loss of consciousness and seizure. He required massive infusions of glucose to reverse this.

REDUCING HYPOGLYCEMIA RISK

Insulin is considered a high-alert medication, meaning there are serious repercussions to taking insulin too liberally. A carefully calculated dosage is key during glycemic control interventions. Taking in more insulin than you need can lead to low blood sugars and hypoglycemia. This is a state in which there is not enough glucose in the bloodstream to meet the body's energy demands. As aforementioned, taking metformin together with insulin and specialized regimens of insulin can mitigate some of these risks. This also highlights the importance of titrating and calculating insulin doses.

In more extreme cases, hypoglycemia starts to affect the brain and central nervous system leading to comas and seizures. In the 1940s and 1950s, insulin shock therapy or insulin coma therapy was popularly performed as a psychiatric treatment for schizophrenia. Some psychiatrists even claimed an 80% success rate. A subsequent study performed in 1957 that compared insulin shock therapy to barbiturate-induced unconsciousness disproved these claims.

LIMITATIONS OF HANDLING, DISPENSING, AND STORING INSULIN

There are a variety of insulin products that may cause patient harm if mixed up. To add another layer of complexity, one can even have different formulations of insulin for the same brand insulin product. One of the limitations of insulin therapy is the fact that frequent regimen changes and adjustments have to be made in the management of diabetes. This means that sometimes the calculations have to be very precise or else there could be serious repercussions. Lastly, there are also some problems that can happen from improper storage of the insulin. Insulin products have unique refrigeration requirements, meaning the insulin must be at a proper temperature prior to administration for it to have the desired effect. Medication incidents have been reported as a result of accidentally leaving the insulin outside of the fridge.

DOES CHRONIC INSULIN USE RESULT IN INSULIN RESISTANCE?

Ironically enough, too much insulin in the blood may actually result in a decrease in insulin sensitivity. Exciting new work in mice models are being conducted to distinguish between primary hyperinsulinemia and secondary hyperinsulinemia. Primary insulinemia is merely a result of an increased concentration of insulin such as from exogenous insulin treatment. This is in contrast to secondary hyperinsulinemia which can occur from a high-glycemic load diet and other metabolic complications like obesity, high cholesterol, and diabetes.

In real patients, these effects are hard to parse out and remain the subject of greater investigation. Nevertheless, it is important to consider that there may be some effect of insulin on developing insulin resistance especially for augmentation therapy where there may still be some residual endogenous insulin function.

CONVENTIONAL MODEL

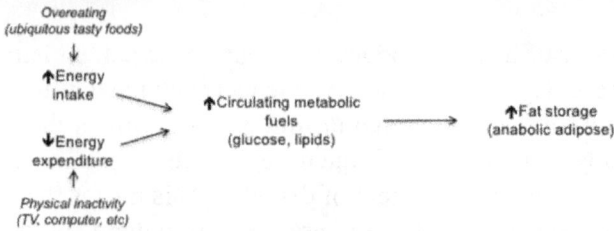

Overeating
(ubiquitous tasty foods)
↓
↑Energy
intake   ↑Circulating metabolic
                              fuels   ↑Fat storage
↓Energy   (glucose, lipids)   (anabolic adipose)
expenditure
↑
Physical inactivity
(TV, computer, etc)

CARBOHYDRATE-INSULIN MODEL

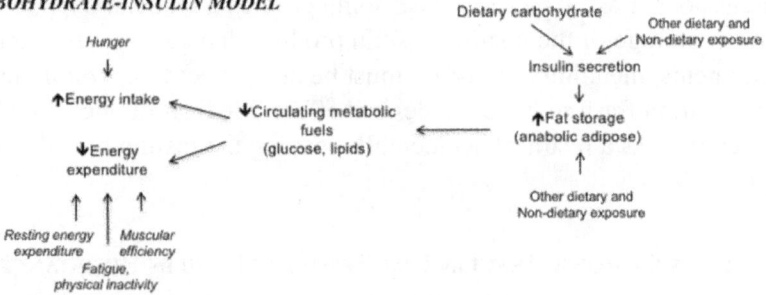

                                        Dietary carbohydrate
                                                              Other dietary and
Hunger   Non-dietary exposure
↓   Insulin secretion
↑Energy intake ←   ↓Circulating metabolic   ↓
                            fuels   ↑Fat storage
↓Energy   ←   (glucose, lipids)   ←   (anabolic adipose)
expenditure   ↑

↑   ↑   ↑   Other dietary and
Resting energy │ Muscular   Non-dietary exposure
expenditure   efficiency
Fatigue,
physical inactivity

Figure 4: Comparison of the 2 theories: 1) Conventional Model and 2) Carbohydrate-Insulin Model of Metabolic Syndrome. [8]

In fact, the Carbohydrate-Insulin Model has been postulated to explain obesity and the ensuing metabolic syndrome as a consequence rather than a cause of increased weight with respect to adiposity. This new model, when juxtaposed with the conventional idea of "calories-in, calories-out." The model suggests that rising blood insulin levels after a meal can push calories to fat cells instead of using it for energy consumption. In turn, this can signal endocrine mediators that increase hunger and slow metabolism, leading to increases in weight and the sequelae that lead to insulin resistance. It should be noted that these ideas are still relatively recent (within the last decade) and based on work-in-progress of experimental rodent models that still need to be validated in controlled human populations. [8]

FINAL THOUGHTS

Insulin is a highly effective and versatile medication that can be used in various regimens for meeting glycemic targets, managing hyperkalemia, reversing growth hormone deficiencies, and enhancing performance to name a few applications. It is important however to be cautious of the potential adverse effects of insulin therapy including the negative effects on the central nervous system that ensue from hypoglycemia as well as the emerging role insulin augmentation therapy may have in causing insulin resistance.

CHAPTER 7
WHICH DELIVERY OF INSULIN IS BEST?

Anthony Chen

Advancements in the development of insulin delivery devices is perhaps just as important as innovations in insulin synthesis or extraction. Insulin administration has evolved significantly since its inception and novel methods of insulin delivery remain as large topics of interest for researchers. When insulin was first made commercially available, it was sold in vials and was administered subcutaneously via syringes (1). Since then, other subcutaneous methods of insulin delivery including computerised insulin pumps and patient friendly insulin pens have been developed. However, all subcutaneous delivery methods suffer from limitations such as risk of infection, patient noncompliance due to pain and fear of needles, induced lipodystrophy (localised fat loss/gain), and local hyperinsulinemia (2). Due to these limitations, noninvasive methods of insulin delivery has been heavily sought after, yet very difficult to develop due to physiological barriers. The first alternative delivery method made commercially available is inhaled insulin which is absorbed through the permeative surfaces of the lungs. However, inhaled insulin has only recently been reintroduced to the market due to controversy in relation to long term lung health (1). Oral insulin is an extremely promising area of development in which several technologies have been put in place to overcome insulin breakdown and absorption barriers within the gastrointestinal tract. Certain oral insulin products are currently undergoing phase 3 clinical trials and will hopefully be commercially available in the near future (3). Buccal, and transdermal (insulin patches) delivery methods are also currently under investigation to evaluate long-term safety and effectiveness (4,5). All insulin products are subject to variations in pricing and availability which heavily informs patients' and physicians' choice. As such, this chapter will aim to explore the various methods of insulin administration and allow readers to assess the best method of delivery for their circumstances.

In the current market, insulin can only be reliably injected subcutaneously (underneath the skin). While recent studies have found that intradermal delivery through microneedling offers faster insulin action, there is currently no available method of intradermal, intramuscular or intravenous injections suitable for periodic self-administration. Subcutaneous insulin injections do not require substantial skill to perform and have been streamlined to be child friendly through modern insulin pens and pumps. The different forms of insulin injections offer various advantages and disadvantages which will be explored in the following sections.

SYRINGES

The earliest syringes used for insulin injections were made of glass and metal, and were reusable. However, after each use the syringe had to be sharpened with a pumice stone and sterilized through boiling, carrying even then a significant risk of infection (1). Insulin syringes have since been modernised and made disposable to reduce the amount of infections and heighten convenience. Modern syringes are marked in insulin units, 30, 50, 100 and 200 U, which correspond to 0.3, 0.5, 1.0, and 2.0 ml capacities (6). This allows for variation in dosage based on patient assessment to be easily prescribed. Some modern insulin syringes include "engineered sharps injury protection" which reduces the risk of injuries during injection. When properly trained, most adults and children at sufficient development levels will be able to self-administer insulin through syringes without significant discomfort (7).

Withstanding, many considerations must be made before using an insulin syringe. While modern syringes are often prepared with bacteriostatic additives that inhibit bacterial growth on skin, needles should still never be reused to avoid infection. Additionally, modern needles of small gauge can be easily deformed which can cause injuries such as lacerations or leave needle fragments stuck in the skin. Lipodystrophy, which is the localised loss/gain of fat, can occur at injection sites and cause undesirable cosmetic appearances. Peripheral hyperinsulinemia, the abnormally high presence of blood insulin, also occurs at injection sites and has been associated with Tau phosphorylation and ectopic fat accumulation (8,9). To minimize these impacts, it is recommended to alternate injection sites, although this practice may increase variability in insulin absorption between injections (6). Finally, for individuals who have low dexterity, visual impairment, or other physical disabilities, the help of other individuals is needed at each injection and may limit the patient's ability to travel throughout the day.

Syringes are a highly accessible and very frequently used method of insulin administration. In Canada, syringes cost just above 20 CAD for a box of 100. This makes them the cheapest insulin delivery device and is thus preferred by many.

Insulin Pen

 The first insulin pens were manufactured in 1985 and since then, they have developed in order to address several of the problems presented with vials and syringes. Modern insulin pen needles are shorter and less invasive, requiring less force to penetrate the skin and less time to inject the insulin. Additionally, pens offer more accuracy and convenience compared to patient prepared syringes, and prevent mistakes in preparation and administration (10, 11). Several studies have found that pen use is correlated with higher patient adherence, and patients who may feel social stigma associated with syringe use (due to association with drug abuse/sickness) may feel more comfortable with pens (12). All of these factors contribute to overwhelming patient and nurse preference for insulin pens when price is not accounted for (13). Commercially available insulin pens include refillable pens such as: Autopen 24, HumaPen MEMOIR, Novopen 4, and OptiClik as well as disposable pens such as: FlexPen, Humalog Pen, and SoloSTAR (10). Some pens include additional functions. For instance, the HumaPen MEMOIR records the time, date, and dosage of each injection for monitoring. In fact many modern pens include smart features such as bluetooth connectivity for logging doses, and built in calculators (7).

Even though it has certain advantages, pens are not considered a replacement for syringes due to their higher prescription costs while achieving very similar therapeutic effects. It has been found that patients switching from syringes to pens show no significant improvement in glycemic control (10). In one study, it has even been found that patients who switched to pen injections displayed deteriorated glycemic control after 5 years (although this could very well be the natural effect of disease progression) (14). Of course, the invasive effects of injection: risk of infection, lipodystrophy, and peripheral hyperinsulinemia remain whether a pen or a syringe is used. All while the cost per unit insulin of pens is generally higher than that of syringes, and additional fees are required for needle replacement. For patients who need to mix insulin formulations, pen use may be less convenient as multiple

47

injections are required. For users of single insulin preparations, the choice between pen and syringe ultimately comes down to how much affordability is valued versus quality of life.

Insulin Pumps

Insulin pumps are computerized devices which deliver insulin through cannula (flexible plastic tubing) to a subcutaneously inserted needle. The first insulin pumps were developed during the 1960s but they were large and non practical. Modern insulin pumps have become very compact and wearable on a belt or in a pocket. A basic insulin pump delivers continuous subcutaneous insulin infusion (CSII), in which a continuous but low basal dosage of insulin is delivered. However, when a patient eats, the pump can also deliver a higher bolus dosage (15). CSII pumps more accurately mimic normal insulin physiology, in which insulin is secreted continuously from the pancreas but secreted at higher rates during meals. This more physiologically similar method of insulin delivery has been found to be important in maintaining basal insulin levels and preventing damage to the eyes, kidneys and nerves (16,17). While multiple daily injections of insulin can also be used to achieve normal glycemia, this method is associated with more extreme glycemic variation and can thus impact patients' quality of life. Many studies have demonstrated that CSII pumps more effectively lowers glycated hemoglobin levels and requires lower insulin dosages in comparison to multiple daily injections (16). In modern CSII pumps, multiple basal infusion rates can be selected from by the patient based on their activity thus allowing patients to be more mobile and flexible with diet and exercise.

More recently, sensor-augmented insulin pumps, which involve communication between pumps and separate blood glucose monitors, have become a reality. The readings from glucose monitors are used to inform the infusion rates of insulin pumps and thus deliver more physiologically appropriate insulin responses (7). Studies have shown that sensor-augmented insulin pumps are even more effective at reducing glycated hemoglobin levels when compared to regular CSII therapy (18). Another advantage of sensor-augmented pumps is that they are able to reduce the likelihood of nocturnal hypoglycemia through the low glucose suspend feature. When blood glucose drops below a threshold rate, insulin delivery is suspended to lessen the severity of hypoglycemia. Some pumps even have predictive low glucose suspension, in which insulin delivery is suspended 30 minutes prior to a predicted hypoglycemic event. In some trials, predictive low glucose suspension has been shown to reduce the rate of nocturnal hypoglycemia by 50-80% (19). One popular choice of insulin pump for Canadians is the Medtronic Minimed 670G which includes predictive low glucose suspend features.

Despite their therapeutic superiority, insulin pumps still have many disadvantages that make them lose patient favor. Most notably, the cost of insulin pumps make them a hefty investment, with the Minimed 670G priced at around 6000 CAD for a yearly subscription on their website. Glucose sensors must also be purchased separately, and thus this upfront cost proves unaffordable for many patients. Furthermore, as pumps involve the continuous use of needles, the risk of infection is also increased and patients must be trained in maintaining hygiene and sterility. To an unwary patient, a detached needle or disconnected device presents a higher risk of diabetic ketoacidosis thus creating more need for patient training (7). Finally, some patients may find carrying a pump to be inconvenient in certain situations such as showering. However, some modern "patch pumps" such as the Omnipod resolve this problem by attaching directly to the skin and communicating wirelessly to a separate monitoring system.

MICRONEEDLING

As mentioned, intradermal insulin administration is not commercially available, but prospects for this delivery method are positive. In trials where insulin is delivered intradermally through microneedles, type 1 diabetic patients demonstrated reduced time for insulin absorption with less variability between administrations. Some rationales for the advantages of intradermal injection explain that higher vascular uptake is achieved from dermal capillaries, or that lymph vessels transport intradermally injected insulin to the circulatory system (20).

One problem presented in microneedling therapy is that patients reported more pain when compared to regular subcutaneous injections. However, this may be due to less developed pain reduction technologies on the microneedling devices used in experimental trials (20). Ultimately, as microneedling advances, it could become an alternative, potentially less invasive and more efficient, method of insulin administration.

INHALED INSULIN

There have only ever been two inhaled insulin products that have been made commercially available: Pfizer's Exubera released in 2006, and MannKind's Afrezza released in 2014. Lung surfaces are much more permeative than gastrointestinal walls and in comparison to orally ingested insulin, inhaled insulin is not subject to breakdown by gastrointestinal enzymes. For these reasons, inhaled insulin became the first prospective non-invasive alternative to subcutaneous injections.

The first inhaled insulin, Exubera, was a powder to be inhaled using a dry powder inhaler. It demonstrated similar effectiveness in lowering glycated hemoglobin in both type 1 and type 2 diabetics when compared to regular injections (21, 22). It could be prescribed in 1 mg or 3 mg doses individually or in combination with longer-acting insulin. However, Exubera was associated with many health risks and was thus contraindicated in several groups. Patients who were smokers or have recently quit smoking, as well as patients with lung conditions such as asthma demonstrated decreased glycemic control on Exubera (21). Additionally, many respiratory side-effects were reported, such as coughs, lung infections, pharyngitis, and even lung cancer. In some trials, patients taking Exubera showed greater pulmonary function decline in comparison to patients with a placebo (23). Ultimately, these factors in combination with its higher cost caused Exubera to lose patient/physician favour and be withdrawn from the market in 2007.

Afrezza is also a dry powder, but the inhaler used for its delivery is much more compact and portable. Clinical trials found that Afrezza shows similar glycated hemoglobin reduction in comparison to regular insulin injections in type 1 and type 2 diabetics, with a reduced rate of hypoglycemia in type 1 diabetics and increased rate of hypoglycemia in type 2 diabetics (1). Unfortunately, the safety concerns associated with inhaled insulin are still very prevalent. Among the side effects are: coughs, long term decline in pulmonary function, increased incidence of lung cancer, and increased risk of bronchospasm in patients with chronic lung disease (7). In general, the introduction of a growth hormone like insulin to the lungs is subject to controversy amongst patients and physicians, and patients should be well informed before being given an Afrezza prescription. Afrezza can cost many times more than competing insulin brands depending on the method of purchase. Of course, with inhaled insulin, the invasive effects of subcutaneous injections are fully avoided, so Afrezza is the only commercially available alternative for patients with concerns about injections.

Oral Insulin

Oral insulin is another non-invasive alternative therapy which has great potential. Oral delivery not only completely eliminates the need for needles, but more accurately mimics the physiology of regular insulin production with insulin travelling from the liver to the rest of the body rather than being distributed from some periphery. Delivery of insulin through the liver has been proven to be more effective than subcutaneous delivery in maintaining appropriate insulin concentrations and controlling hepatic glucose output (3). For type one diabetics, oral insulin may have the potential to induce an "oral tolerance", in which the immune system becomes less avid in disrupting β-cells in the pancreas. This can delay disease progression and suppress autoimmune diabetes, but has only been successfully demonstrated in mice (24). For type two diabetics, oral insulin allows for "β-cell rest", in which the secretion of insulin from the pancreas is suppressed. β-cell rest has been correlated with improved insulin secretion and β-cell viability and can diminish the progression of disease if oral therapies are initiated early (25). Generally, oral insulins are a much more convenient product which more accurately corrects the physiology of diabetics.

However, oral insulin is very difficult to develop due to the conditions of the gastrointestinal tract. Insulin as a protein hormone is broken down by protease enzymes such as pepsin, trypsin, carboxypeptidase, and pancreatin during digestion. Ultimately, the purpose of the digestive system is to break down larger molecules for absorption and it does so indiscriminately. Additionally, undigested insulin can not be absorbed through gastrointestinal walls. The epithelial cells of the villi, lining the intestines are tightly bound and are covered by a layer of mucin protein which prevents the passing of large polymers (3). To bypass the conditions of the digestive system several technologies have been incorporated in oral insulin products. For instance, some oral insulins are delivered with protease inhibitors such as sodium glycolate. Other oral insulins are PEGylated (bonded to polyethylene glycol chains) which makes the molecule more stable and has been shown to increase insulin absorption as well as facilitating prolonged insulin action (26). Another promising method is the use of permeation enhancers such as bile salts to increase the permeability of epithelial cells and thus the absorption of insulin (27). Most recently, some oral insulins have been encapsulated using nanoparticles in alginate microgels. This protects the insulin from digestive enzymes and furthermore, the nanoparticles have been developed so that they are able to pass epithelial cells through small masses of lymphatic tissues in the small intestine (Peyer's patches). This method of producing oral insulin has been successful in controlling blood sugar in mice but has not entered clinical trials (28). Many of these technologies are novel and must be tested for long-term side effects. For instance, protease inhibitors have the potential to disrupt digestion and permeation enhancers could cause damage to the gastrointestinal walls (3).

Some oral insulin products such as IN-105 and Capsulin, which involve PE-Gylation and permeation enhancers, are currently undergoing phase 3 clinical trials. If these drugs become approved, it is not unreasonable to assume that oral insulin may eventually hold a large share of the insulin market.

Buccal Insulin

Buccal insulin refers to insulin that is absorbed through the buccal mucous membrane. Theoretically, the buccal mucous membrane has an extensive network of blood vessels which should allow for rapid absorption of insulin. Unlike the inner membrane of the lungs, the buccal membrane is exposed to constant trauma from eating, and thus there is less chance of long term damage. However, like epithelial cells, the buccal lining is not very permeative to large molecules. Buccal insulin products thus combine a variety of additives that allow the insulin to pass the membrane through intercellular space. Buccal insulin is found in liquid form and delivered using an asthma puffer like device called the RapidMist system (4). In type 1 diabetics, buccal insulin induces a higher a faster rise in blood insulin than when subcutaneously injected, although blood insulin would also drop faster thereafter (4). Buccal insulin is somewhat effective in reducing glycated hemoglobin and this has been demonstrated in multiple studies (29). However, more trials are necessary in order to gauge the long-term effectiveness and safety of buccal insulin. One buccal insulin product, Oral-lyn, is currently available in India, but is still undergoing phase 3 trials in the US. and Canada.

Transdermal Insulin

Transdermal administration transports insulin across the skin using minimally invasive methods. One advantage this allows over oral, inhaled, or buccal deliveries is that continual release similar to CSII can be achieved (5). Evidently, skin is impermeable to large proteins and as such, several technologies have been developed to facilitate the absorption of insulin transdermally. These include: chemical enhancers that increase skin permeability, Iontophoresis to drive charged insulin to the capillaries through electrostatic forces, ultrasounds to induce cavitation in the skin, and jet injections which fire high speed insulin containing streams into the skin (5). While there are currently no reliable products, transdermal insulin is a developing field in which promising results are being found regularly.

Conclusion

Insulin administration is a field of many prospects, and it is very possible that in the near future, a novel method of insulin delivery will be deemed the safest, least-invasive, and most practical method. However, at the moment, it is necessary to choose between different health risks at different price points. It is thus important for patients to evaluate their own circumstances in choosing the most appropriate method of insulin administration.

CHAPTER 8
HOW AND WHERE IS INSULIN PRODUCED IN THE BODY

April Sui

The general process of making insulin involves transcription of the needed genetic material, synthesis of the protein and finally the secretion of mature insulin. At each point, diverse regulatory events from within our body as well as other physiological factors will influence how and where insulin is made. This chapter aims to explore the mechanism and location of insulin production in the human body.

GENES AND TRANSCRIPTION

The production of insulin begins with the information needed to encode this protein in our DNA. The gene coding for insulin in humans is located on the shorter arm of chromosome 11 (2). The exact locus of the gene will differ among mammals, though it is expressed exclusively in the β-cells of the pancreas. For humans, the insulin gene (Figure 1) contains two introns and three exons (2).t

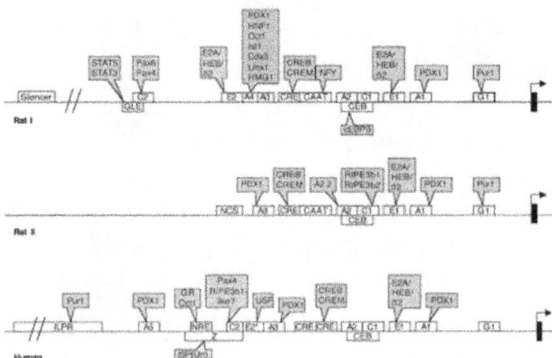

Fig. 1. Enhancer and promoter regions for human, rat I and rat II insulin (3 p310).

The first of three steps in the transcription of DNA into RNA in eukaryotes is initiation. The section of DNA containing the insulin gene is unwound and transcription factors bind to a region on the promoter (1). Inside the nucleus, RNA polymerase II is recruited and the transcription factors are released, allowing for synthesis of the new strand to start (1). The second step is elongation, where RNA polymerase moves along the DNA template strand and synthesizes RNA by adding nucleotides (1). The new strand grows from 5' to 3' and is antiparallel to the template strand (1). Lastly, termination of the transcription occurs when the complete RNA strand is released and the DNA strand returns to its original helix shape (1).

Regulation of transcription is important in maintaining normal production of insulin. In particular, gene expression is restricted to β-cells of the endocrine pancreas, ensuring tissue specificity. This is controlled by regulatory regions flanking the 5' end (2,3).

Various other elements of the insulin gene such as the A, E, and C elements in Figure 1 are involved in regulatory processes (2). The proteins that bind to each sequence are also presented above each box and play crucial roles.

Positive regulation implies events leading to the activation of insulin gene transcription, such as with an activator or enhancer (2). Regulatory cis-acting elements and trans-acting factors are involved in insulin gene transcription (2,3). Insulin genes share numerous conserved DNA sequences in the regions flanking the 5' end (3). This suggests a possibility that these genes are regulated by similar trans-acting factors (3).

In particular, the E boxes (E1 and E2 in Figure 1) bind to basic helix-loop-helix proteins, or bHLH proteins (3). These are potent transcriptional activators of tissue-specific genes which then interact with BETA2 and NeuroD, regulatory proteins synthesized in neuroendocrine and pancreatic cells (3). Studies have found that the E box is able to differentiate between varying bHLH factors when binding in order to attain accurate tissue-specific gene activation (3).

Though effective on their own, the individual elements on the insulin gene can also produce synergism through collective interactions (2,3). Multiple activators operating on a single complex of the insulin gene allows for combinatorial control. This grants the ability to employ more than one regulatory input into a single output (3). Such cooperative interaction has been studied between the proteins that bind to E and A elements (3). PDX-1, a factor binding to A3 and A4 elements (Rat I of Figure 1), works in synergy with E47 from the bHLH transcription factor family (3). This phenomenon requires DNA binding and activation domains of the PDX-1 and bHLH proteins (3).

Negative regulation involves a silencer that decreases gene expression (3). BETA3, a B class specific bHLH that is closely homologous to BETA2 and NEUROD, is a negative regulator of the E box (3). BETA3 can not bind to the E box despite its own intact basic region. Thus, it inhibits E47 from binding to DNA and represses the transactivation of insulin enhancer that is mediated by E47 and BETA2 (3). The activity of other proteins associated with the E box is influenced by this, as well as the synergism it brings about involving A element-binding proteins (2,3).

Id proteins and c-Jun transcription factors associated with E elements also play a role in negative regulation. Id proteins belong to the helix-loop-helix (HLH) family and lack basic domains for binding DNA, thus lowering binding affinity to DNA (3). The most evidence found regarding its function is with inhibiting rat II insulin promoter activity when high glucose exposure causes it to be overexpressed (3). The c-Jun transcription factor creates inhibition by acting through E1 (3). The result is repressed transcriptional activation caused by the basic leucine region on c-Jun (3). Similarly, c/EBP beta is another member of the leucine zipper family of TF that represses gene transcription specifically in β-cells by targeting the enhancer (3).

Studies have found upregulation in β-cells that faced chronic levels of exposure to glucose and in models conducted using diabetic rats experienced downregulation of insulin expression (3). Thus, it appears that glucose metabolism is also a major physiological regulator of insulin expression in the body (3,4).

Post-transcriptional regulation of insulin controls the stability of the insulin transcript and affects protein production (2,4). Glucose plays a key role in maintaining the stability of insulin mRNA after it has been transcribed from DNA (2,4). Studies conducted in in-vitro conditions found that insulin mRNA stability decreased when exposed to lower glucose concentrations and increased with higher concentrations of glucose (2). When glucose is not present in β-cells, insulin mRNA levels undergo a sharp decrease that is reversed by increase in intracellular cAMP levels (2).

Translation concerns the assembly of amino acid polypeptides on ribosomes to synthesize a protein (1). For eukaryotic cells, this process occurs mostly in the cytosol and consists of 3 steps (1). During initiation, the ribosome is formed from its subunits and scans along the mRNA until it recognizes an AUG start codon at its P site as seen in Figure 2 (1). A methionine-tRNA with the corresponding anticodon pairs with it and any protein initiation factors are released (1). Elongation involves synthesizing the polypeptide chain . An aminoacyl tRNA will bind to the A site on the ribosome. Peptidyl transferase then cleaves the amino acid from the tRNA in the P site and creates a peptide bond linking it to the amino acid on the tRNA occupying the A site (1). In Figure 2, this action is exemplified as a methionine (Met) amino acid is bound to phenylalanine (Phe) to form a polypeptide chain. The ribosome translocates forward along the mRNA from 5' to 3' and the tRNA that shifts to the E site is released before the process is repeated (1). Finally, termination occurs when the mRNA's stop codon (UAG, UAA, UGA) reaches the P site (1). Release factors bind to the A site and stimulate peptidyl transferase to cleave the finished polypeptide at the P site in order to release it (1). The

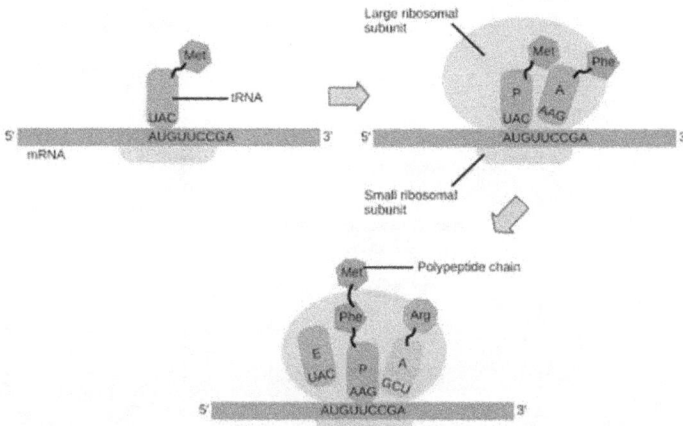

Fig.2. The process of elongation in translation (5).

release factors and tRNA are released and the ribosomal complex separates from the mRNA (1).

When the insulin mRNA is translated, the resulting product is not mature insulin. Rather, translation synthesizes insulin's precursor; a highly conserved, single-chain molecule of 110 amino acids known as preproinsulin (2,3). Preproinsulin then undergoes post-translational modification (Fig.3) to remove the central segment of amino acids while leaving the insulin molecule, two polypeptide chains (A-chain and B-chain of Fig.3) linked by disulfide bridges, intact (2,6).

First, the hydrophobic N-terminal signal peptide sequence on preproinsulin interacts with ribonucleoprotein signal recognition particles (SRP) found in the cytosol (2,6). SRPs facilitate the movement of preproinsulin across the membrane of the rough endoplasmic reticulum (rER) and into its lumen (2). Proinsulin is then formed when preproinsulin's signal peptide is cleaved by a signal peptidase (2,6). This new molecule folds and forms three disulfide bonds with the help of various endoplasmic reticulum chaperone proteins (2). When it's three-dimensional conformation has matured, proinsulin is transported out of the ER and to the Golgi apparatus where it enters pre-mature secretory vesicles (2). It is then cleaved to form insulin and a C-peptide, which are kept in secretory granules along with islet amyloid polypeptide, or amylin, and other β-cells secretory products (2).

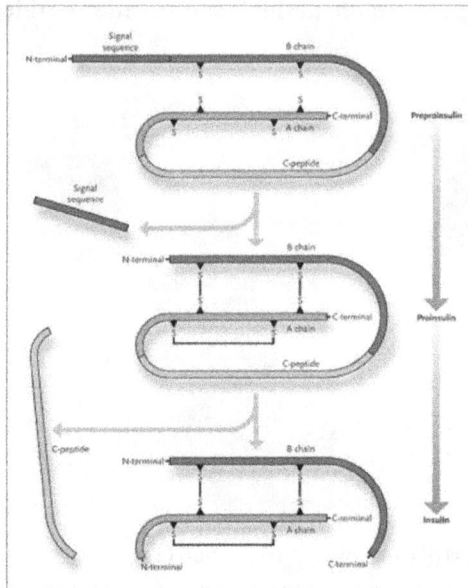

Fig.3. Post-translational modification of preproinsulin (6 p1932).

Similar to the events of gene transcription, the translation of insulin also undergoes regulation. β-cells will enhance their general speed of protein translation in response to nutrients (2). This is partially controlled by dephosphorylation of the eukaryotic initiation factor 2a (eIF2a) through protein phosphatase 1 (PP1) (2). Research conducted regarding this phenomenon discovered that β-cells experienced a substantial decrease in the ratio between phosphorylated eIF2a and eIF2a after being exposed to high glucose for 2 hours (2). A protein responsible for phosphorylation of eI-F2a is pancreatic ER kinase (PERK), which also occupies a crucial role in regulating translation (2). Mutation of PERK resulting in abnormal function can give rise to defective insulin synthesis and medical conditions such as Wolcott-Rallison syndrome (2).

β-cells are also able to regulate the speed of insulin translation to adjust insulin production in response to immediate environmental triggers. One study of rat islets concluded that exposure to 25 mM glucose over the course of 1 hour resulted in increased intracellular proinsulin levels by up to ten times the baseline level (2.8 mM glucose), all while proinsulin mRNA quantities remained constant (2).

Furthermore, β-cells have a mechanism in place to identify the amount of insulin that is stored and secreted and the cells will adjust synthesis accordingly (2). This feedback control involves islet cell autoantigen 512 (ICA512), a granule transmembrane protein (2). Insulin granules travel on tubulin tracks to reach the peripheral actin network and are attached to the actin cortex by ICA512 and β2-synthrophin (2). The granule is then connected to the cytoskeleton. When the granule is activated, the membrane of the granule will fuse with the cell membrane in order to release insulin via exocytosis (2). In the meantime, the cytosolic fragment from ICA512 is cleaved off by the protease μ-calpain which is activated by increased Ca^{2+} ion levels (2). The free ICA512 fragment then moves in the cytoplasm to the nucleus where it binds to STAT5, a tyrosine-phosphorylated transcriptional factor (2,3). This binding keeps STAT 5 from being dephosphorylated and effectively upregulates the transcription of insulin (2). Free ICA512 cytosolic fragments found in the nucleus will also bind to PIASγ, a sumoylating enzyme that then sumoylates the ICA512 (2). This undoes the binding of ICA512 to STAT5, creating positive feedback as the successful release of insulin from secretory granules is related to the nucleus (2).

SECRETION AND DISTRIBUTION

Following the synthesis of complete insulin, the protein is then secreted from the cell. β-cells of the pancreas secrete insulin into areas of the pancreas known as islets of Langerhans (1). These are formed by endocrine cells, which make up about 2% of all cells found in the pancreas (2).

The secretion of insulin by exocytosis is a process that involves many different proteins. N-ethylmaleimide-sensitive factor attachment protein receptor (SNARE) is soluble and responsible for the fusion of an insulin granule to the plasma membrane (2). A β-cell exocytotic core complex is created when four SNARE motifs come together to form a stable helical structure (2). The four SNARE motifs also contribute four highly conserved amino acids to the complex's central portion (2). This group is made up of one arginine (R) residue and three glutamine (Q) amino acids (2).

The formation of another complex also partakes in the fusion of the insulin granules with the plasma membrane for β-cells. The required components are syntaxin-1a (Qc-SNARE) on the plasma membrane, VAMP-2 (R-SNARE) on the granule membrane as well as the membrane-associated protein SNAP-25 (Qa-Qb SNARE) (2). In order to successfully regulate the insulin granule fusion, other accessory factors may also become involved in the assembly process of the complex. For example, the regulatory factor Tomosyn-1, which is capable of replacing VAMP2, can be present during assembly (2). A lack of Tomosyn-1 produces no effect on insulin transport and docking, however, this factor is still required for the fusion and sometimes priming of granules (2).

A clear biphasic pattern is exhibited in insulin secretion; it consists of a transient first phase followed by a more constant second phase (2). In humans, when plasma glucose is around 7 mM, the first phase of insulin secretion peaks at 1.4 nmol/min (2). The first phase lasts for approximately 10 minutes and is then followed by the second phase with the secreting rate at about 0.4 nmol/min (2).

Insulin granules resulting from translation and post-translational processing can be divided into two categories based on their mode of function. A small fraction of the granules are immediately available for release. The readily releasable pool (RRP) comprises 1% of the total granules and contributes to the rapid release of insulin triggered by the presence of glucose (2). The reserve pool is made up of the remaining 99% of granules. When the RRP is exhausted, granules from the reserve pool replace the lost ones (2). These must first undergo preparatory reactions, a priming process that includes translocation toward the plasma membrane and granule modifications. It also happens to be the rate-limiting step in insulin exocytosis (2).

There is evidence to suggest a relationship between insulin secretion's biphasic pattern and the different granule pools. Both exocytosis from the RRP and the first phase of insulin secretion can occur even in conditions where nutrients are absent (2). Meanwhile, RRP granule replacement and the second phase of insulin secretion are both strictly dependent upon metabolic products (2). There is also a positive correlation between the total number of granules in RRP and the amount released during the first phase of insulin secretion (2). The removal of Munc13-1, a diacylglycerol receptor, suppresses specifically insulin granule exocytosis as well as second phase insulin secretion (2). However, it has no effect on insulin exocytosis from the RRP or the first phase (2). Withstanding, there remains a kinetic discrepancy in that RRP replacement is relatively fast, happening in 1 second, compared to the first phase of secretion that can endure around 10 minutes (2).

Priming and fusion of the granules resulting in insulin exocytosis is triggered by elevation in levels of intracellular Ca^{2+} concentration (2). Exocytosis is carried out at a rate of 500 granules per second when intracellular Ca^{2+} concentrations are increased to 17 mmol/L and proceeds at 3–4 granules per second when concentrations are at 0.17 mmol/L (2). Exocytosis will still happen at low Ca^{2+} concentrations because a small portion of granules are capable of releasing insulin in such conditions (2). These are known as the high Ca^{2+}-sensitive pool (HCSP) (2). The different rates of exocytosis are controlled by two mechanisms for sensing Ca^{2+}; the lowaffinity Ca^{2+} sensor and the high affinity Ca^{2+} sensor (2). At high Ca^{2+} concentrations, the ongoing exocytosis is controlled by the low affinity Ca^{2+} sensor. An example of a high-affinity Ca^{2+} sensor is synaptotagmin IX, observed in β-cells and the subject of study concerning its true function (2). One possibility is that it can also work similarly to a low-affinity Ca^{2+} sensor (2).

Piccolo is another type of putative Ca^{2+} sensor that interacts with essential proteins in order to facilitate rapid Ca^{2+} induced exocytosis (2). It has interactions involving cAMP-regulated guanine nucleotide exchange factor, sulfonylurea receptor1 (SUR1) along with L-type Ca^{2+} channels (2). This suggests the possibility that piccolo can act as a low-affinity Ca^{2+} sensor (2). The regulation of insulin secretion greatly involves the nutritional state of the cell (2,3). β-cells are capable of detecting change in plasma glucose concentrations and respond by releasing appropriate amounts of insulin (2). β-cells are found clustered in islets that are purposefully connected to the vasculature, forming a dense network with small blood vessels (2). Thus, the islets receive 10 times the amount of blood that cells in the surrounding exocrine regions would receive (2). Capillaries that surround the islets possess a considerable quantity of fenestrae (2). These small pores facilitate greater nutrient exchange between the circulating blood and the surrounding tissues , and improve permeability (2). With unrestricted nutrient access, β-cells can sense the nutritional state quickly (2). The enhanced permeability also allows for the swift diffusion of insulin into the bloodstream (2).

An example of a hormone that regulates the secretion of insulin by the pancreas glucose-dependent insulinotropic peptides (GIPs) (2). The secretion of this hormone increases with the presence of glucose in the duodenum, triggering the release of insulin (2). This usually happens when blood glucose levels are high. Contrarily, when blood glucose levels are low, β-cells are not stimulated and insulin secretion decreases (2).

The production of insulin in the human body as well as its various regulation mechanisms continues to be studied. Findings provide further insight into the causes and potential treatments of disease originating from abnormal insulin production, such as forms of diabetes.

CHAPTER 9
ALTERNATIVES TO INSULIN FOR DIABETES TREATMENT AND MANAGEMENT

Nasia Sheikh

Insulin is one of the most common treatment options for patients with type 2 diabetes, and the sole treatment option for type 1 diabetes (1). The primary goal for type 2 diabetes treatment is to lower blood glucose levels (2). Insulin has been used as a treatment for diabetes to reduce blood glucose levels since 1922, and in recent decades, through countless research studies, various forms of insulin treatments have been developed in an effort to increase efficacy and safety of patients (1). Insulin treatment, however, can often have side effects such as, hypoglycemia – low blood sugar, and cause excessive weight gain (2). Individuals with diabetes may also find injecting themselves repeatedly uncomfortable.

Typically, treatment of type 2 diabetes begins with lifestyle changes; however, if these changes are not sufficient in managing diabetes then treatments move to oral anti-diabetes medications (2). If oral anti-diabetes medications are also unsuccessful, then insulin treatments are used. Aside from direct insulin treatment, there are many other types of non-insulin medications used to treat type 2 diabetes (3).

METFORMIN

Metformin is an oral anti-diabetes (OAD) medication and is typically the first OAD medication prescribed to type 2 diabetes patients (2). Metformin falls under the biguanide class of medications which have been used to treat diabetes mellitus for decades (4). Biguanides typically have antihyperglycemic properties, which is mainly a consequence of reduced glucose output due to inhibition of liver gluconeogenesis and to a lesser extent, increased insulin-mediated glucose uptake in skeletal muscle (4).

Metformin, in earlier years, was considered weaker than other glucose-lowering biguanides, thus they were not used as widely (5). As a result, other forms of glucose-lowering biguanides including, phenformin and buformin, were used primarily instead. However, the uses of such medication were withdrawn in the late 1970s due to links to side effects such as lactic acidosis. Continued research in the 1980s and 1990s demonstrated the uniqueness and importance of metformin to manage hyperglycemia, therefore it was not withdrawn as a treatment option (5).

Metformin is now the primary OAD used to treat type 2 diabetes and has been shown to lower glucose levels as well as improve insulin sensitivity (4). Despite being the most frequently prescribed anti-diabetic treatment worldwide, its mechanism of action is not well understood.

Looking at the history of Metformin, its herbal lineage can be traced back to Galega officinalis, more commonly known as French Lilac, or professor weed, which is a traditional medicine used in medieval Europe (5). G. officinalis is known to have benefits against epilepsy, fever, and in 1772, John Hill recommended Galega to treat "conditions of thirst and frequent urination" which is now recognized as a common indicator of diabetes (5). When chemically analyzed, G. officinalis was found to contain high levels of guanidine, which was reported to reduce blood glucose in animals. In the 1920s, several mono-guanidine derivatives were also shown to lower blood glucose in animals; however, they were associated with high levels of toxicity, which effectively diminished their use as a diabetes treatment (5).

The fusion of two guanidines to form biguanide in later research provided the origin of metformin (5). Biguanides were reported to lower blood glucose levels and were less toxic than mono-guanidines; however, high doses were required to achieve effective glucose lowering results (5). This led to biguanides, including metformin, being pushed aside for more promising diabetic treatments such as insulin.

During the 1980s, with exploration into non-insulin-dependent diabetes, metformin became a drug of interest again, as a trademark of this type of diabetes was insulin resistance, and metformin was known to counter insulin resistance (5). Studies in the 1980s and early 1990s demonstrated that the ability of metformin to reduce hepatic gluconeogenesis and increase peripheral glucose utilisation was not only an result of respiratory-chain disruption, rather it affected a number of insulin-dependent and independent effects. These effects varied in different tissues based on overall drug exposure and nutrient metabolism within these tissues. Of importance, it was highlighted that high levels of metformin in the intestinal walls have insulin-independent effects, which is responsible for excess lactate production while in the liver and muscle tissues, there are lower concentrations of metformin which alter post-receptor insulin signalling pathways and redirect energy-generating and storage pathways (5).

The primary effects of metformin are seen in the liver, where it inhibits gluconeogenesis by blocking a mitochondrial redox shuttle (6). However, the effects of metformin are pleiotropic, as metformin has also been shown to be an insulin sensitizer and likely acts in the gut lumen through various mechanisms (6). Despite the vast knowledge of some of the effects of metformin and its long history in medicine, the exact mechanism of action remains elusive. Despite this, it is frequently prescribed as treatment of hyperglycemia in patients who have type 2 diabetes and its use is supported by sixty years worth of clinical studies (6).

THIAZOLIDINEDIONES (GLITAZONES)

Thiazolidinediones (TZD) are a class of drugs used in the treatment of type 2 diabetes mellitus as an insulin sensitizer (7). There have been numerous TZDs throughout history that have been explored and used as a treatment for diabetes. In 1975, Japanese based laboratories synthesized numerous analogues of a lipid-lowering agent called Clofibrate and discovered that some of the analogues demonstrated hypoglycemic effects in diabetic mice (7). In 1982, the first TZD, Ciglitazone, was discovered and showed promising lipid and glucose lowering effects in animal models (7). Unfortunately, it resulted in liver toxicity and was therefore discontinued (7).

In 1988, Troglitazone was discovered, which showed potential glucose lowering effects and was later approved by the FDA for type 2 diabetes treatment in 1997 (7). Unfortunately, 6 weeks after approval, it was withdrawn from market due to a rare but potentially fatal hepatotoxicity (7). At the same time, two other potent insulin sensitizers called Rosiglitazone and Pioglitazone were being developed and were later approved by the FDA for management of type 2 diabetes (7). Both of these drugs were reported to not be toxic on the hepatic system, but Rosiglitazone was later shown to increase cardiovascular risk and Pioglitazone was shown to have increased risk for bladder cancer (7). Thus, restrictions were placed on prescribing both Rosiglitazone and Pioglitazone.

The primary purpose of TZDs is to control hyperglycemia in type 2 diabetes patients by lowering the fasting blood glucose levels and reducing the concentration of the glycosylated form of hemoglobin (7). This reduction in insulin resistance is accomplished by enhancing insulin sensitivity in muscle cells, adipose tissue, and possibly hepatic cells (8). However, the exact mechanism of action of TZDs is unknown.

The molecular mechanisms of the biological response of TZDs that are understood are believed to be mediated through the modulation of Peroxisome Proliferators Activated Receptors (PPARs) (7). PPARs are a group of nuclear receptor proteins that regulate the expression of genes, specifically they function as transcription factors. These receptors are reported to be involved in multiple pathways involved in metabolism thus making them important targets when managing a metabolic syndrome (7). TZDs have also been shown to possibly enhance beta-cell function, which has implications for maintaining long term glycemic control in type 2 diabetes (9).

TZDs also possess a number of advantages. TZDs are cheaper than newer diabetic treatments such as Exenatide, Glargine, and Detemir and are similar in cost to insulin regimens (7). TZDs have also been shown to reduce urinary excretion of albumin and other proteins as well as interferes with the development and progression of diabetic neuropathy (7).

Overall, the use of TZDs in the management of type 2 diabetes is well established, but further research is required into the mechanism of action.

INCRETIN BASED THERAPIES

Many long term complications of diabetes have a background of chronic inflammation. Incretin hormones have hypoglycemic properties and a history of anti-inflammatory effects, thus they have potential in treating and managing diabetes (10).

Incretin based therapies were first developed in the 1960s after discovering that incretin signals originating from the gut increased cell response to caloric intake and that gut hormones play an important role in the physiological response to glucose (11).

It has been shown that there is an increase in stimulation of insulin secretory responses from oral glucose administration compared to intravenous administration (12). This is referred to as the incretin effect; release of incretin hormones and their insulinotropic action on pancreatic cells in response to glucose (12). Essentially, the incretin effect defines an interaction of gut signals with the pancreas.

Incretin hormones typically have low basal plasma concentrations and are released after eating and increase the insulin secretory response (12). There have been two peptides synthesized and secreted from the gut that have been identified as incretin hormones: glucose-dependent insulinotropic polypeptide (GIP) and glucagon-like peptide (GLP-1) (12). In healthy individuals, it is believed that GIP and GLP-1 production increases in response to oral glucose intake, effectively increasing the production of insulin to maintain glucose levels.

It is believed that the incretin response in type 2 diabetes is defective. This defective incretin response is also likely to determine the pancreas's ability to secrete insulin in response to oral glucose (eg food ingestion), therefore, contributing to hyperglycaemia in type 2 diabetes patients (12). This highlights the importance of the incretin effect for maintenance of normal glucose levels.

Incretin based therapies are targeted at lowering glucose levels by restoring the incretin effect. Common incretin based therapies include exenatide and sitagliptin (10).

BARIATRIC SURGERY

Pathophysiological connections between diabetes and obesity have long been recognized. It has even been stated to likely be "the biggest epidemic in human history" (13). Millions of people have diabetes, and even larger populations have obesity. Obesity is thought to be one of the strongest risk factors for development of type 2 diabetes (13). This makes sense when exploring the biology of both diseases. Obesity is associated with various pathophysiological changes that increase insulin resistance (13).

These diseases, especially in combination have negative implications on quality of life, mortality, and morbidity (13). Treating individuals with diabetes and obesity is important not only for the health improvements of the individuals, but also in terms of reducing burden on the healthcare system.

Typically, the first mode of action when diagnosed with diabetes, is lifestyle changes often targeted at weight loss; however, obese individuals with diabetes tend to have more difficulty reducing weight compared to individuals without diabetes (13). Therefore, therapeutic options to reduce and maintain weight is required. One such treatment is Bariatric surgery.

Bariatric surgery is a type of weight loss surgery and can lead to remission of diabetes. Following surgery, glycemic control is restored by a number of mechanisms including, enforced caloric restriction, enhanced insulin sensitivity, and increased insulin secretion. Slight improvement in glycemic control was expected following weight loss from the bariatric surgery, however, there was a secondary, surprising observation as well. The immediate post-surgical glycemic improvement suggested short-term mechanisms of action that were separate from long-term mechanisms (13). The effects of bariatric surgery on diabetes have been explored further in research.

In addition to glycemic improvement following bariatric surgery, some patients also experienced improvements in insulin sensitivity, a crucial component of diabetes pathogenesis, to a similar extent as patients who lost a similar amount of weight through caloric restriction (13).

Exploring patients who underwent bariatric surgery also illustrated evidence that the gut microbiome may contribute to improvement in glucose homeostasis (13). It is unclear if the gut microbiome was altered due to metabolic improvement, or if there was metabolic improvement due to substantial changes in the gut microbiome. Regardless, studies show that the gut microbiome is markedly altered following bariatric surgery, with an increase in microbiome diversity (13).

Perhaps the most striking result of bariatric surgery in diabetic patients, is that the rapid improvement in glycemic control precedes weight loss (13). Some case reports show that patients who had pre-surgical insulin requirements were insulin-free at the time of discharge. It is believed that this is due to alterations in gut hormones (13).

Although bariatric surgery may seem like a drastic treatment option, there are many benefits to the procedure and may result in remission of diabetes in some patients. Other treatment options such as lifestyle modification and intensive medical therapy may also result in better control or even remission of type 2 diabetes, but many patients find it difficult to achieve sustained control of blood glucose (14). Intense medical therapy can also lead to hyperglycemia and weight gain (14). Bariatric surgery may be the best option available to some patients due to a myriad of physiological, behavioural, and financial barriers preventing them from accessing more conventional therapies (13).

ARTIFICIAL PANCREAS

The primary goal in treatment of type 1 diabetes is maintaining good glycemic control without hypoglycemia (15). Despite many advances in medicine and technology, this still presents with many challenges for both patients and healthcare providers (15). The most common current treatments for type 1 diabetes is multiple daily insulin injections or continuous subcutaneous insulin infusion by an insulin pump (15). Some studies have shown that the continuous insulin infusion had more favourable effects on glycemic control in type 1 diabetes patients compared to multiple daily injections (15). However, both of these treatments can be very taxing on patients. Repeatedly injecting oneself multiple times a day can be very difficult as well as painful and can cause skin damage and fat and scar tissue to build up. The subcutaneous insulin infusion by an external insulin pump can also be very cumbersome after an extended period of time. They also require continuous glucose monitoring systems to ensure correct amounts of insulin are being administered, which needs to be manually adjusted thus can be very time consuming (16).

Aside from the two above-mentioned treatments for type 1 diabetes, a less common emerging treatment is the artificial pancreas treatment, also referred to as closed loop glucose control. This treatment combines an insulin pump and continuous glucose monitoring with a control algorithm to deliver insulin in a glucose responsive manner (15). There are also dial hormone artificial pancreas systems where glucagon is also delivered in a similar glucose responsive form (15).

With the artificial pancreas treatment, there is a reduced burden for patients, as the amount of insulin entering the body becomes automated based on glucose level sensors (15). There have also been numerous studies validating the use of an artificial pancreas and its efficacy and safety (15).

In conclusion, there are many alternatives to insulin treatments for both type 1 and type 2 diabetes. Each comes with their own unique set of advantages and disadvantages and may not be ideal for every patient. There are a myriad of factors that need to be considered when choosing diabetes treatments, and although one may be an excellent choice for one patient, it may not be for another.

Research into diabetes treatment and management, however, is continuous and widespread, which will hopefully result in even more efficient and safe treatments in the future.

CHAPTER 10
CONSPIRACY THEORIES ABOUT INSULIN

Arnavi Patel

INTRODUCTION

Insulin therapy has been shown to be an effective treatment for diabetes, however, patients oftentimes refuse it. There are many barriers that patients may face when making the decision to start insulin therapy. Some common barriers include fears of hypoglycemia, needles, restricted lifestyle, and organ damage (1, 2). Further, misconceptions and fears held by physicians can also create barriers for patients to receive insulin therapy. Physicians are sometimes hesitant to provide insulin therapy to patients because they feel they have failed their patients in controlling their diabetes, and often do not want to force their patients on a troublesome regime (1, 2, 3). In this chapter, misconceptions and fears regarding insulin therapy will be explored. Further, the current available research regarding some misconceptions will also be addressed. Lastly, possible methods to address patient concerns and physician concerns will be discussed.

PATIENT FEARS AND MISCONCEPTIONS ACT AS BARRIERS TO INSULIN THERAPY
THE FEAR OF NEEDLES

The fear of needles is often felt when considering insulin therapy. This fear can be further divided into three parts, painful injections, self-injections, and a phobia of needles (2). Patients currently on insulin therapy report needles are often painful (2). This can play a major role in deterring many considering patients away from pursuing this treatment. Second, patients also have negative feelings regarding administering needles themselves. Some say they are uncomfortable with watching themselves get needles and are often apprehensive of self injecting (2). Third, many people have a phobia of needles (2). Fears can often cause many people to avoid certain activities.

71

Diabetes patients with a fear of needles may have trouble administering
needles on a daily basis, because their fear may interfere.

The Fear of Restricted Lifestyle and Stigma

Further, patients also feel insulin may interfere in their daily lives and cause
embarrassment or stigma (2). Many feel insulin therapy is an inconvenience
and often impractical (2). Patients on insulin therapy also have to maintain
fitness through exercises and monitor their diet, which can feel restricting
(2). Lastly, patients feel there is a stigma around insulin therapy as some
may equate it to drug use (2). Patients also feel they are not confident
enough to handle needles and insulin therapy (2).

The Fear of Hypoglycemia

Hypoglycemia is a common experience among patients taking insulin
therapy, causing some to have this fear when considering insulin therapy.
The fear of hypoglycemia is a widespread fear (4). According to Frier et
al (2015)., there are many factors that are linked to this fear. These factors
include a history of hypoglycemia, the length of insulin therapy, and a(?)
variability in blood glucose level (5). While hypoglycemia can occur from
insulin therapy, it is common for patients to have mild episodes which
do not warrant immediate medical care (5).Frier et al (2015)., show on a
weekly average Type 1 diabetes patients experience 2.4 non-severe events
of hypoglycemia, and Type 2 diabetes patients experience 0.8 non severe
events of hypoglycemia (5). According to the results of the study, 26% of
these events occurred during the night, and 20% of these events caused interference in work life for those who were working at the time (5). However,
patients almost never informed their healthcare providers of these events (5).
This study found non severe hypoglycemia is common among adults taking
insulin therapy (5). This study shows hypoglycemia is a normal occurrence
for patients on insulin therapy, however oftentimes the risk is not severe.

In the event that a patient is likely to experience hypoglycemia with insulin
therapy, there is an alternative that may help. The risk of severe hypoglycemia can be reduced with the use of insulin lispro (6). Insulin lispro is similar
to human insulin however, the proline and lysine in positions 28 and 29 in
the C-terminus of the B chain are in opposite places (7). Insulin lispro also
has faster rates of absorption and glucose-lowering activity (7). Studies
show the risk of episodes of hypoglycemia is lower with lispro insulin (7).
In one study, 4.4% of participants using regular insulin experienced an episode of hypoglycemia whereas only 3.1% of participants using insulin lispro

experienced an episode of hypoglycemia (7). Hypoglycemia can possibly occur when taking insulin therapy, however mild cases are common and alternatives to regular insulin are available to reduce the risk of severe cases.

THE FEAR OF ORGAN DAMAGE

Another frequent fear patients have is organ damage due to insulin (5). Kidney damage has been linked to insulin resistance from the body (8). Resistance to insulin causes an increase in production and secretion of compensatory insulin from the pancreases which can lead to hyperinsulinemia to maintain euglycemia (8). If the insulin secretion cannot be adequately increased to overcome the insulin resistance, hyperglycemia and glucose intolerance can occur (8). Insulin resistance and glucose intolerance has been linked to kidney diseases (8). Further, glomerular hyperfiltration and increased vascular permeability are induced by hyperinsulinemia (9). This plays a role in kidney dysfunction, and is associated with insulin resistance (9).

One of the causes for insulin resistance is Angiotensin II (Ang II) (10,11,12,13,14,15). Ang II is a major effector hormone of the renin-angiotensin system (RAS) which plays a major role in the maintenance of vascular and renal homeostasis (13). Ang II also has an effect on insulin receptors, insulin receptor substrate proteins, the P13-Kinase/Akt pathway, and GLUT4 (13). Two insulin receptor substrates that are affected by Ang II are IRS-1 and IRS-2 (14). Ang II is thought to stimulate tyrosine and serine phosphorylation of IRS-1 and IRS-2 (14). These substrates are known to bind to the P13-Kinase (14). Ang II inhibits insulin stimulated IRS-1 and IRS-2 associated P13-Kinase activity by stimulating the serine phosphorylation of the insulin receptor β-subunit in IRS-1 and the p85 regulatory subunit in the P13-Kinase (14). This causes interference with the docking of IRS-1 with the p85 regulatory subunit of the P13-Kinase, which results in inhibition of insulin stimulated IRS-1 associated P13-Kinase activity (14). Insulin is able to carry out its function of maintaining the transportation of glucose into the cell through a series of steps involving the P13-Kinase (16). Activation of the P1k-Kinase occurs when insulin binds to IRS-1 (16). Disruption in this series of events causes insulin to not be able to do its job correctly, thus causing insulin resistance (16).

Insulin resistance can lead to further complications. Inhibition of insulin associated activity by Ang II is also linked to many major cardiovascular risk factors (10). Studies show there is a significant relationship between imparied insulin action and cardiovascular disease (10). Ang II and insulin

73

resistance is implicated in the path to cardiovascular disease (10). Further, aldosterone, a hormone part of the Renin-Angiotensin-Aldosterone system (RAAS), has also been connected to insulin resistance and cardiovascular disease (11). This hormone is linked to defective intracellular insulin signalling, impaired glucose homeostasis, and insulin resistance in skeletal muscles, the liver, and cardiovascular muscles (11). The negative effects of RAAS on insulin sensitivity is mediated by the activation of Ang II and receptor type 1 (AT1R) and increased production of mineralocorticoids (11).

However, research shows there are some treatments to lessen the effects of Ang II and aldosterone on insulin inactivity. By blocking Ang II and AT1R Insulin resistance and cardiovascular disease morbidity and mortality are decreased, and glucose homeostasis can be increased (11). Further, oral administration of Ang II receptor antagonist Irbesartan also effectively increases insulin activity (15). Ibersartan increases glucose tolerance and insulin mediated glucose transport in the epitrochlearis and soleus muscles (15). Glucose tolerance increases due to an enhancement in skeletal muscle glucose transport (15). A dose dependent increase in insulin action is predominantly seen in type I soleus muscles (15).

FEARS AND MISCONCEPTIONS OF PHYSICIANS AS BARRIERS TO INSULIN THERAPY

Some misconceptions and fears are also helped by physicians which prevent patients from receiving the care they need. Before starting insulin therapy, patients often use oral agents. If oral agents do not continue to work for patients, physicians sometimes feel they have failed their patients in control of their diabetes (3). For this reason, physicians are reluctant to recommend insulin therapy to diabetes patients. A study in Nigeria looked at perceptions of general physicians about insulin to determine barriers to insulin for patients (1). They found the most common barrier to insulin therapy is fear of hypoglycemia (1). Results show, 81.3% of respondents say they are hesitant to start insulin therapy for patients due to fear of hypoglycemia (1). The second most popular reason for recommending insulin therapy was fear patients will reject it (1). This concern was followed by concerns regarding pain from needles (65.6%), insulin storage (59.4%), and affordability (57.8%) (1). Some physicians are also resistant to starting insulin therapy due to the lack of confidence in themselves to initiate it (1).

However there are steps physicians and researchers can take to help ease these fears. Research shows physicians should listen to patient concerns and support them through the process (2). If physicians do not have confidence in starting insulin therapy for their patients, it can cause patients to hesitate more. Patients who have their doctor's emotional and physical support are more likely to initiate insulin therapy (2). Further physicians may also try to threaten patients with insulin therapy (17). This is done to encourage patients to continue maintaining their diabetes without insulin therapy (17). However, this is a barrier for many patients as insulin therapy can help maintain and control their diabetes. Treatments that patients are on before switching to insulin therapy may not work the same as they used to (2). Denial of insulin therapy from physicians prevents patients from receiving the best care for their diabetes. Many physicians and patients also believe insulin therapy should be a last resort in the event that oral therapies do not work (1). However this mentality only prevents diabetes patients from receiving the best care. Research shows patients who are educated about insulin therapy, as well as the myths and misconceptions surrounding insulin therapy, are more likely to pursue it (2). Providing patients with education and information regarding insulin therapy is the necessary next step to addressing fears and concerns.

FACTORS TO ACCEPTING INSULIN THERAPY

Some factors that helped patients accept insulin therapy are the limited benefits of oral treatments, learning that insulin is natural, and the belief that insulin improves health, maintains glycemic control and prevents complications (2). Patients say they switched from the oral treatments to insulin therapy because oral treatments ceased to work (2). After a while oral agents are no longer effective in maintaining blood glucose level. Further, learning that insulin is natural to the body also eases the fears and uncertainty around insulin therapy (2). Patients are more likely to inject something they know is natural. Moreover, patients say they switched to insulin therapy because it provides a better quality of life (2). Patients also say they feel more energetic when taking insulin (2). Further, patients take insulin to reduce the risk of amputation and dialysis (2). Information regarding insulin therapy is usually obtained through searching the internet, talking to relatives, and reading material regarding information about the insulin therapy (2). An accessible method of delivering information regarding insulin therapy is crucial in combating misconceptions surrounding the treatment.

To address myths and misconceptions about insulin therapy, Bord et al (2014)., created a tool for patients. First the authors considered the major questions diabetes patients would like to address (17). Participants in the study were asked what the key barriers to accessing insulin treatment were. These included long term complications from the therapy, possible side effects of the therapy, inconvenience of treatment, fear of needles, and possible weight gain from insulin, and the beliefs that insulin is a last resort treatment, and a failure to self manage diabetes (17). Participants were also asked the best way to receive educational information regarding insulin. Results show participants want a tool that is accessible and easy to understand with neutral unbiased facts from trusted sources and perspectives from patients (17). The authors created a brochure style tool with carefully researched answers to popular questions from participants (17). In a cognitive debriefing, the language was assessed to ensure it was clear, understanding, inoffensive, and relevant, and the format was acceptable (17). After four blocks of cognitive debriefing, minor revisions were required before it was accepted (17).

Tools such as the one created by Brod et al (2014)., are important for diabetes patients considering insulin therapy. Patient perspectives are as equally important as facts. Testimonies from patients helps other patients who may be hesitant or apprehensive to feel more comfortable with starting insulin therapy. Further patient testimonies also help physicians to understand who benefits the most from insulin therapy and how to better help diabetes patients. Many patients that start insulin therapy often do research beforehand by reading material online and speaking to relatives and friends. Providing diabetes patients with an educational tool that is catered to them will help store a lot of the information in one accessible place. This helps patients gather information regarding insulin therapy easily leading to ease of concerns. Patients will also be able to make an informed decision as they will know about the possible outcomes, and side effects of insulin therapy from trusted sources and other patients. Patients may trust information presented on an accessible tool, if it addresses their needs well.

FUTURE DIRECTIONS

Going forward, educational tools for patients and physicians regarding the misconceptions about insulin therapy should be developed. These educational tools are essential for informing patients about insulin therapy. With these educational tools any questions and concerns that patients may have will hopefully be answered. Moreover, educational tools provide patients with a sense of comfort regarding insulin therapy. It is important to be transparent about insulin therapy and provide patients with the consequences and benefits. This will help patients gain trust in healthcare providers and trust in the treatment itself. Further, patients will be able to make an informed decision whether or not they want to start insulin. Educational tools for physicians should also be developed. These tools should include ways to listen to patient concerns and assess cases carefully. Physicians should be aware of the misconceptions surrounding insulin therapy as well as patient perspectives. Further, physicians should be provided adequate resources and training to support patients through insulin therapy. With the implementation of these educational tools, there may be less fear and misconceptions regarding insulin therapy.

CONCLUSION

In conclusion, there are many reasons why patients may refuse insulin therapy. These include fear of needles, the belief that insulin therapy is for severe cases of diabetes, fear of organ damage, fear of hypoglycemia, and fear of a restricted lifestyle among others. Some physicians are also apprehensive to give insulin therapy to patients as they believe insulin therapy should be used as a last resort for diabetes treatment or they feel they have failed in treating their patients with self management and oral agents. However, these act as barriers which prevent patients from receiving the best care possible. Insulin therapy has many benefits for diabetes patients, however due to these misconceptions these benefits may be overlooked. The best way to help diabetes patients is by providing education and support. Education helps patients make informed decisions about insulin therapy by taking into account the negatives and positives. Support is also necessary for patients undergoing insulin therapy because they may not feel comfortable with starting it. In the future with developments for education and support, diabetes patients may not feel so apprehensive about insulin therapy.

CHAPTER 11
EMERGING EXPERIMENTAL RESEARCH AND THE FUTURE OF INSULIN THERAPY

Peter Anto Johnson

EMERGING EXPERIMENTAL RESEARCH
UPPER GI TRACT INSULIN CHEMOSENSING

Insulin and other neuro-endocrine mediators are present throughout the digestive system. The opening to the gut is the oral cavity which houses the tongue and upper esophagus, the central sites of chemosensation in the upper gastrointestinal tract. Taste transduction is located in the taste buds of the tongue papillae (1), within pharyngeal and laryngeal chemosensory clusters (CCs) and in other gut regions (2, 3). It should be well noted that only taste receptors found in taste buds are associated with the sensory gustatory system and contribute to the taste perception while other taste receptors sites utilize visceral sensation. Each of the five taste modalities: sour, salty, bitter, sweet and umami have specific pathways innervated by the facial (VII) and glossopharyngeal (IX) cranial nerves. (4)

RECEPTOR-LEVEL PROCESSES

At the receptor-level, various processes detect and transduce chemical signals into electrical waves of depolarization transmitted from taste cells to sensory afferents (SAs) (1,5), which lead to cranial nerves VII and IX. Generally, taste cells can be classified into Type I (glial-like) cells, Type II (receptor) cells, and Type III (presynaptic) cells. In addition to the specific roles of these cell types, they have all been suggested to play some role in taste transduction. For example, it is postulated that the Type I cells are the sites for detecting salty taste. Various Na+ channels on the taste bud apical membrane and epithelial Na+ channels (ENaC) promote entry of Na+ ions into the membrane after NaCl dissociates in saliva causing depolarization of the cell membrane and subsequent Ca2+ influx. The transmitter release mechanism, which is not known (1, 4), then activates SA fibers. Since glial cells do not receive direct synaptic innervation by SAs, the mechanism probably involves paracrine action. All of these transduction mechanisms are implicated in the release of insulin from the pancreas due to the presence of the taste signal.

SIGNAL TRANSDUCTION MECHANISMS

Type II receptor cells play a significant role in the detection of sweet, bitter and umami taste which utilizes a more complex transduction mechanism involving G-protein coupled receptors (GPCRs). The general mechanism follows the Gq transduction pathway, involving an isozyme of phospholipase C (PLC) that catalyzes breakdown of phosphatidylinositol 4,5-bisphosphate (PIP2) to diacylglycerol (DAG), and inositol trisphosphate (IP3). IP3 is the ligand for ligand-gated Ca^{2+} channels in the endoplasmic reticulum membrane containing calcium stores causing intracellular Ca^{2+} to increase. As a result, there are two outcomes: TRPM5, a Ca^{2+}-dependent and taste-selective cation channel is activated resulting in a strong depolarizing current and a gap junction hemichannel pore, composed of Panx1 subunits, opens as a result of both high levels of intracellular Ca^{2+} and depolarization enabling release of ATP and presumably other molecules (4, 6). ATP activates ionic P2X receptors on SAs transmitting an impulse to gustatory cranial nerves. It can also have autocrine and paracrine effects by acting on P2X/P2Y receptors on the receptor cells and presynaptic cells, respectively. Autocrine excitation generally increases ATP production while paracrine presynaptic excitation has a limiting effect via the release of serotonin (5-HT), inhibiting Type II cells from producing ATP. This allows for regulated potentiation and confinement of signaling ATP within a defined and localized space.

Specific chemosensing mechanisms for sweet, bitter and umami differs at the level of the type of GPCR and which subunits activate the pathway. There are two main families of taste GPCRs: T1Rs associated with umami and sweet tastes and T2Rs associated with bitter tastes. It is important to recognize Type II cells have further subtypes as sweet, bitter and umami taste-specific cells (1, 4-9). For sweet taste ligands, the $G\alpha$ subunit activates PLC whereas bitter tastants activate $PLC\beta2$ isozyme with the $G\beta\gamma$ subunits (10). Sweet Type II cells contain T1R3 homodimers and T1R2/T1R3 heterodimer GPCRs for artificial sweeteners and sugars while T2R GPCRs detect bitter tastants including PROP and denatonium. While sweeteners follow the general mechanism, sugars activate the Gs pathway by activating adenylyl cyclase increasing cAMP, which activates protein kinase A (PKA) that phosphorylates and inhibits K^+ channels resulting in inhibition of hyperpolarization hence depolarization. Depolarization then raises intracellular Ca2+, releasing neurotransmitters. On the contrary, the bitter taste transduction is suggested to follow a Gi pathway as the α-subunit of the G-protein, gustducin, activates phosphodiesterase (PDE), catalyzing the breakdown of cAMP and cGMP. In bitter Type II cells, cAMP and cGMP normally inhibits cNMP-inhibited Ca2+ channels. When cAMP and cGMP is reduced, Ca2+ influx is promoted and ATP and other neurotransmitters are released via Panx1 pores. In the case of umami tastes, the T1R1/T1R3 binds L-amino acids particularly L-glutamate found in monosodium glutamate (MSG) in noodles and meat broth using the same mechanism as T2Rs (7, 11-13). Based on studies with mouse taste buds, Horio et al. suggests these channels may be TWIK1/2, TREK1/2, or TASK1 channels (6). ENaC were once held to play a role in the uptake of extracellular H+, however it appears to have lost support over the years. This may be a result of gene knockout experiments in mice (1, 6, 14), which indicate various subtypes of these channels were not necessary for sour taste detection. Depolarization causes Type III cells to release 5-HT and perhaps other excitatory molecules into the SA synapse by vesicle release. Once SA fibers are excited, they carry information to cranial nerves VII and IX.

VISCERAL PATHWAYS

Several visceral pathways are also present in the oral cavity and pharynx (13, 18). While molecular chemosensing mechanisms are proposed to involve a similar mechanism to bitter Type II taste cells with the α-gustducin Gi pathway and Gq pathway involving TrpM5-mediated depolarization, the cells found in CCs excite vagal (cranial nerve X) afferent fibres instead of SA fibres. CCs have been identified in the epiglottis, pharynx, larynx, and areas in the superior esophagus. (17, 19)

LOWER GI TRACT CHEMOSENSING MECHANISMS

In addition to perceived gustatory mechanisms, there are also several autonomic or visceral mechanisms that detect chemical substances causing salivation, anorexigenic effects that reduce hunger, gut secretions, peristalsis or segregation, release of hormones like insulin, metabolism of nutrients, and other interesting responses. Recent research has gained much momentum in considering chemosensing via insulin and other mediators in the oral cavity and supraesophageal region of the gut, enteroendocrine cells (EECs) are the primary transducer cells found in the stomach and intestines that detect contents in the gut lumen responding by synthesis and secretion of signaling molecules that have endocrine or paracrine effects.

Insulin directs carbohydrate metabolism and biosynthesis. By the time carbohydrates arrive at the sites of carbohydrate chemosensing in the gut, they have already been broken down to monosaccharides by amylases and brush-border enzymes. Of these monosaccharides, glucose is the most ubiquitous molecule and may be detected in the gut by a number of different mechanisms. One of the generally accepted models of glucose chemosensing in EECs, particularly the L and K cells, is electrogenic Na+-coupled glucose cotransport via SGLT-1 which causes sufficient inward current for membrane depolarization and consequent voltage-gated Ca2+ influx resulting in endocrine release of incretin hormones. (13) Incretins function to lower blood glucose by acting on pancreatic β-cells of the islets of Langerhans stimulating insulin release, inhibiting glucagon release and activating the satiety center to reduce food intake. (12, 14) As such, incretins have therapeutic uses in treatment of diabetes. It has also been suggested that GLUT2, a facilitated glucose transporter, could possibly play a role in this model although inhibition of these transporters by antagonists suggest they are not necessary for glucose chemosensing. (13) These transporters work by expediting the aggregation of glucose within EECs and partaking in glucose metabolism, which activates glucokinase, a crucial enzyme in glycolysis. Due to glycolysis, the electron transport chain and various ATP-producing pathways in the cell, there will be a high intracellular ATP/ADP ratio and the action of weak inwardly rectifying ATP-dependent K+ (KATP) channels will be inhibited. (12) Inhibition of KATP channels prevents hyperpolarization enhancing depolarization of the L or K cell activating voltage-gated Ca2+ channels and allowing for release of the incretin hormones: GLP-1 and gastric inhibitory peptide (GIP), respectively. 5-HT acts on 5-HT3Rs on extrinsic vagal afferents causing reflex gastric motility inhibition and pancreatic secretion, which allows emptying of stomach content and breakdown of chyme. (14) An alternative hypothesis to glucose sensing, proposes that T1R2/T1R3 are responsible for incretin release. (12, 13, 19) The molecular mechanism of chemosensing follows the mechanism for sweet taste receptors found in Type II taste cells. In this case however, glucose replaces the sugar as the ligand and the released transmitters are the incretins. This hypothesis is presently disputed, since knockout of T1r2 gene (coding for T1R2 GPCRs) in mice had no significant influence on normal homeostasis. (13, 19)

There are also hypothesized pathways for monosaccharides other than glucose. For example, galactose is sensed by replacing glucose as a substrate in the SGLT-1 pathway (14) and fructose uses GLUT5 as a facilitated transporter in a mechanism similar to the GLUT2-glucokinase-KATP channel mechanism (13). Nonetheless, chemosensing mechanisms for these mono-saccharides are currently still poorly understood. Insulin is recognized to play a stimulatory role in these processes nonetheless.

L-AMINO ACIDS, PEPTONES, AND PROTEINS MECHANISMS

Insulin has an effect on protein metabolism that takes place detached from the transport of glucose or amino acids into the cell, glycogen synthesis, and the stimulation of high energy phosphate formation. In fact, most proteins are formed in the absence of insulin although insulin does lead to a net generation of protein. Following proteolysis in the stomach and degrada-tion of protein structures in the intestine, L-amino acids, dipeptides and tripeptides are common products, which are detected by chemosensing. L-amino acids generally involve mGluRs, T1R1/T1R3 found in Type II umami cells, $Ca2+$-sensing receptors (CaRs), associated with extracellular $Ca2+$ sensing, and a GPCR subtype (GPRC6A). (12) Nakamura et al. (11) has described L-glutamate sensing activates gastric enterochromaffin cells to release 5-HT activating 5-HT3Rs on vagal afferents causing motility inhibition in the stomach and secretions in the duodenum similar to glu-cose. GPRC6A seems to act by a Gi and Gq mechanism similar to Type II bitter taste cells. It is more prevalent in gastric parietal cells and sense basic amino acids like L-lysine and L-arginine. (12) This could play a role in pH regulation within the stomach. CCK increases bile secretion by gall blad-der contraction, stimulates pancreatic enzyme secretion, and activates the satiety center, which may be useful for treating obesity. In contrast, the CaR is coupled to a Gq mechanism that senses aromatic L-amino acids such as L-phenylalanine, L-tyrosine and L-tryptophan in L cells. Using L-glutamine as a prototypical amino-acid, another mechanism employs $Na+$-amino-acid electrogenic cotransport which follows the same mechanism as the electro-genic SGLT-1-mediated glucose mechanism with SGLT-1 replaced by the amino-acid specific cotransporter, several of which have not been identified.

Less is known about chemosensing and chemical transduction of hydro-lyzed protein products and the role of insulin. It is clear, however, that CCK release is increased by L cells and that G cells in the gastric antrum detect increased pH, luminal $Ca2+$ and proteolytic products and respond to these chemical signals by increasing endocrine gastrin release to promote muco-sal growth and increase HCl acid secretion by parietal cells in the stomach corpus. (12) Busque et al. (2, 12) has suggested CaR on G cells may be re-sponsible for this response, exceptionally when oligopeptides or amino acids are co-perfused with $Ca2+$ in the lumen, which is consistent with its role as an extracellular $Ca2+$ sensor. Another more recent proposal by Rettenberger et al. (16) is that LPAR5 (GPR92/3), a peptone-detecting GPCR has a high expression level in G cells. This GPCR acts by Gq and G12/13 mechanism, the latter more involved in cellular effects like stress fiber formation than hormone release. (9) LPAR5 plays a major role in peptone-detection in the intestine mucosa and has also been described to promote CCK transcription and release in L cells. Similarly, PEPT1, an H+-coupled oligopeptide cotransporter has these same effects when it senses oligopeptides. It follows the same chemosensing mechanism as electrogenic SGLT1 and L-amino-acid transporters with the exception that the initial inward current is generated by H+ influx. PEPT1 and CaR are expressed primarily in intestinal I cells promoting the actions of CCK in response to proteolytic products. Conversely, peptones show not only these effects as they also induce GLP-1 release by STC-1 and NCI-H716 cells, sites of EEC differentiation in the small intestine and colon, respectively. (12, 13)

Free Fatty Acids (FFAs) Mechanisms

Insulin has a fat-sparing effect. The degraded products after lipolysis of lipids by lipases in the small intestine are acyl glycerols and fatty acids including SCFAs, medium chain fatty acids (MCFAs) and long chain fatty acids (LCFAs). EECs contain several Gq-coupled GPCRs activating transmitter release through a Type II cell-type mechanism that detect unsaturated MCFAs and LCFAs. These include: FFAR1 and GPR120 (FFAR4), which are found primarily in small intestine I, K and L cells releasing CCK, GIP and GLP-1, respectively. Along with GIP's role in insulin and glucagon release, it should also be noted to play a crucial role in fat metabolism and activation of adipocyte lipoprotein lipases. On the other hand, SCFAs are sensed by FFAR2 and FFAR3 expressed predominantly in the colon where gut microbial colonies aggregate facilitating fermentation and metabolic processes ultimately generating SCFAs like formate, acetate, propionate, and butyrate as end products. While FFAR2 is Gq/Gi-coupled like T2Rs, FFAR3 is Gi-coupled, operating by cNMP-inhibited Ca2+ channel activation. Both of these receptors are found on enterochromaffin cells involved in vagal afferents. Another prominent lipid sensing mechanism involves Gs-coupled GPR119 (same as Type II sugar mechanism) found in K and L cells that detect the LCFA oleoylethanolamide and monoacylglycerols, products of triglyceride hydrolysis. SCFAs and MCFAs also result in release of neurotensin, which has roles in dopamine-signaling, thermoregulation, etc., however neither receptors nor transduction mechanism of N cells are known. An understanding of these mechanisms are critical for future design of insulin therapy.

Gut chemosensing mechanisms and pathways are integral to mediate essential responses that function to aid metabolism, nutrient intake and utilization, homeostasis and other vital physiological processes. Chemosensing mechanisms have significant overlap in the oral cavity/pharyngeal regions and gastroenteric regions. The main difference was that taste cells release transmitters to SAs or other taste cells rather than to enteric neurons, vagal afferents, other EECs, enterocytes, or into the bloodstream like EECs. Understandings of these mechanisms have contributed to both our understanding of pathology such as the use of incretins to study diabetes type 2 and therapeutic advancements like insulin and CCK to control obesity. Although extensive progress has been made over the recent years, our understanding of gut and insulin chemosensing is still incomplete with various gaps. An understanding of these mechanisms can directly translate to better therapeutics for disease management. Emerging dimensions of taste physiology, gastroenterology, and enteric endocrinology promise deeper insights into chemosensing mechanisms and evolution of our current knowledge.

FUTURE OF INSULIN THERAPY

Current trends suggest the evolving future of insulin therapy holds promise. In addition to innovations such as new injectable types and formulations of insulin, advancements in the artificial pancreas, recombinant and stem cell therapies, closed-loop technology for tighter glycemic control, and novel routes of insulin delivery including transdermal, inhaled, buccal, and second- and third-generation insulin administration *per os* only touch the surface of developing bodies of experimental and clinical research.

INJECTIBLE FORMULATION

New generation formulations of ultra-long basal insulin analogues similar to degludec and glargine U300 are have offered much promise for control of nocturnal hypoglycemia, with less fluctuations in glucose levels (19). One of these new formulas is peglispro (a combination of lispro insulin and polyethylene glycol). Peglispro functions by decreasing the diffusion time required for insulin, which can increase its duration of action. According to phase 3 clinical trials, peglispro was able to achieve lower HbA1c levels and lower the risk for adverse effects including nocturnal hypoglycemia and less blood glucose fluctuations. However, this formulation had its limitations and was demonstrated to increase transaminase and triglyceride levels, which led to its suspension from development. Nonetheless, this has led to a growing body of research on ultra-long acting basal insulin.

Currently, immune-focused therapies are useful, particularly in type 1 diabetes patients, to prevent or slow the loss of beta cell mass in the pancreas. Of these cell-directed and cytokine-mediated interventions, one novel strategy has involved the use and development of an Fc-conjugated insulin derivative, LAPS-Insulin115, which shows great promise as a candidate for once weekly injections.

Recombinant formulations, which use genetic modifications to insulin, are another avenue under current investigation. Many ultrarapid insulins, which are useful for fast-onset management of postprandial glucose excursions (e.g., FIAsp (insulin aspart + nicotinamide and L-arginine), while already on the market are still problematic for management if delayed. As a result, Insulin-PH20 (rHuPH20) combines both rapid acting insulin and recombinant human hyaluronidase, which leads to interference in hyaluronic acid present in the subcutaneous tissue. This can thereby lead to faster absorption, a shorter time for onset, a better effectual management of postprandial glucose when compared to lispro, as well as a similar safety profile to existing insulin therapies. Another interesting combination is the lispro insulin complex based on BioChaperone technology which brings together polymers, oligomers, and small organic molecules to form a complex that is resistant to enzymatic breakdown, has an increased absorption profile, and bioavailability – all of which enhance its rate of action.

GLUCOSE-RESPONSIVE INSULIN SYSTEMS

Glucose-responsive insulin (GRI) systems or "smart-insulins" are a new generation of insulin therapy that relies on endogenous feedback to sense blood glucose levels. Simplistically, this system is composed of a glucose sensor, which is a compound that can be altered in response, and an insulin delivery system. GRI systems can be classified into two classes: polymer-based systems and molecular GRI systems. The first class - polymer-based systems - make use of glucose-binding compounds to encapsulate insulin into a polymeric vesicle, hydrogel, or other complex that can incorporate lectin, bio-molecules like glucose oxidase, phenylboronic acid, and/or other glucose-binding proteins. The second class of GRI systems directly modifies the insulin formulation through covalent conjugation to phenylboronic acid, enabling the introduction of a glucose-sensing motif in the generated complex. While both classes of GRI systems have been demonstrated for efficacy in animal models, further validation is warranted prior to clinical trials and implementation.

The subcutaneous delivery of insulin has gained a great deal of interest over the recent years with the development of several new technologies and devices. For example, the InPen and other smart insulin pens, which can be paired with Bluetooth, enable dose calculation adjustments, reminders, tracking, and health data monitoring (19). The last decade has been characterized by a spike in the development of mobile apps for enhancing data monitoring and enhancing daily adherence to insulin therapy. Another subcutaneous delivery device is the insulin jet injector, where high pressure air is administered on the skin to avoid introduction of needles in the patient allowing fast onset of action and better postprandial glucose control. Although jet injectors are promising and a variety of jet injectors are on the market, maintenance is tedious and bruising can occur if inadequate pressures are generated. A more recent innovation in the subcutaneous delivery of insulin that has also gained much traction and development are insulin patch-pump systems. Several models of patch-pump systems are already on the market including V-Go, PAQ, Omnipod System, and ePump systems. These technologies are much more discrete, compact, lightweight, disposable or semi-disposable compared to conventional pumps and do not require any tubing. They can be directly attached to the skin by either an adhesive strip or flexible cannula. Nevertheless, the safety and efficacy of these systems must still be assessed in cohorts of diabetes patients to ensure their feasible use as a therapy.

PULMONARY DELIVERY SYSTEMS

Pulmonary administration of insulin offers several therapeutic benefits including an enhanced delivery due to large alveolar and capillary surface area, thin alveolar walls and the absence of insulin-cleaving peptidases in the lung environment that would enhance insulin clearance. As a result, a variety of inhaler technology has been tested in this context. One promising product is Dance-501, which is a compact, pocket-sized inhaler utilizing a vibrating mesh micropump technology and liquid insulin formulation, which is currently in Phase 3 clinical trials (19, 20). Another one is Promaxx, which uses microsphere technology that utilizes a liquid preparation of recombinant human insulin and has a similar total metabolic effect to subcutaneous injections of regular insulin. An even more recent innovation has been Spiros, which is a breath-actuated inhaler that uses aerosolized human insulin powder and allows for a shorter time to achieve the maximum metabolic effect. There are also numerous other emerging devices which make use of nano- or microparticle inhalation for the delivery of insulin through the pulmonary system. Notably, disadvantages with these techniques is the variable bioavailability that can result as a consequence of pulmonary factors, side effects such as cough or an allergic response, and long-term safety, which has not yet been demonstrated.

ORAL INSULIN ADMINISTRATION

Administering insulin as tablets is an existing method of delivery. Products such as GIPET 1, ORMD-0801, CapsulinIR, and Tregopil are all administered per os and available on the market. These tablets are composed of regular insulin or analogues alongside permeation enhancers and/or protease inhibitors (19). In numerous studies, oral insulin formulations have shown hypoglycemic effects in subjects with Type 1 and Type 2 diabetes. Insulin analog tablets, which include Tregopil, also allow for rapid absorption of insulin and effective clearance. Ultimately, enteral delivery routes can not only increase absorption as it has direct access to the portal circulation once absorbed in the gut but also factors such as patient compliance, adherence, and allow for greater convenience. However, it is key to note that insulin is not well-absorbed in its natural state and oftentimes requires additional permeation enhancers and/or protease inhibitors to allow for effective absorption and overcome enzymatic degradation and clearance.

BUCCAL INSULIN ADMINISTRATION

The administration of insulin buccally is another attractive alternative due to the easy accessibility, increased surface area for absorption, enhanced permeability, decreased presence of peptidases, and excellent regeneration and healing after injury. Oral-lyn, MidaForm insulin, PharmFilm are all examples of buccal insulin formulations (19). These are a technology-liquid formulation of human recombinant insulin & absorption enhancers that have more rapid onset of action and faster clearance when using polymeric film embedding recombinant human insulin. Although buccal administration may be a convenient noninvasive route for insulin delivery, more clinical trials and development are necessary prior to its recommendation and implementation clinically. There are also patient factors such as preference, which tends to be lower for this route of delivery, that must be considered.

With the skin being the largest organ in the human body, transdermal approaches have many advantages as an accessible surface for absorption. However, it may also have its limitations, particularly due to its low permeability and increased risk for irritation and allergic reactions (19). As a result, many modern approaches have studied the use of chemical enhancers, iontophoresis, electroporation, sonophoresis, jet injectors, and micro-needle assisted delivery. Chemical enhancers use conventional molecules & membrane-permeable peptides or vehicles to deliver insulin. Methods like iontophoresis and electroporation are coupled to electrical voltage gradients or fields to enhance the permeability of skin, whereas approaches such as sonophoresis and jet injectors are coupled to mechanical processes that improve skin permeability. Micro-needle assisted delivery involves penetrating the skin to create microchannels to facilitate the delivery of insulin. This has been associated with improved absorption and decreased hypoglycemic adverse effects in animal models, which makes it a promising avenue for current research. At present however, more investigation is still crucial to progressing research.

REFERENCES

CHAPTER 1

1. Bliss M. The History of Insulin. Diabetes Care. 1993;16(Supplement_3):4–7.
2. Vecchio I, Tornali C, Bragazzi NL, Martini M. The Discovery of Insulin: An Important Milestone in the History of Medicine. Frontiers in Endocrinology. 2018;9.
3. Hoskins M. Historic Look at Insulin Prices and Access | DiabetesMine [Internet]. Healthline. Healthline Media; 2019 [cited 2021May8]. Available from: https://www.healthline.com/diabetesmine/history-of-insulin-costs#How-It-Used-To-Be

CHAPTER 2

1. Best, C.H. Frederick Grant Banting 1891-1941. The Royal Society Publishing. [Internet] 1942 Nov [Cited 2021 May 7th] 4(11). 20-26 Available from: https://www.jstor.org/stable/769145
2. Canada Land A. Frederick Grant Banting [Internet]. Library and Archives Canada. 2016 [cited 2021May7]. Available from: https://www.bac-lac.gc.ca/eng/discover/military-heritage/first-world-war/100-stories/Pages/banti ng.aspx#a
3. Collip, J.B. Frederick Grant Banting, Discoverer of Insulin. The Scientific Monthly [Internet]. 1941 May [cited 2021 May 7th] 52 (5): 472-474. Available from: https://www.jstor.org/stable/17312
4. Stansfield, W. D. The Discovery of Insulin: A Case Study of Scientific Methodology. The American Biology Teacher [Internet]. 1941 May [cited 2021 May 7th] 74 (1): 10-14. Available from: https://www.jstor.org/stable/10.1525/abt.2012.74.1.4
5. Root-Bernstein, R. Frederick Banting, Painter. The MIT Press [Internet]. 2006 [cited 2021 May 7th] 39 (2): 154. Available from: https://www.jstor.org/stable/20206188

6. Weaver, J. The Discovery of Insulin. British Medical Journal [Internet]. 1984 May [cited 2021 May 7th] 288 (6412): 239. Available from: https://www.jstor.org/stable/29513779

CHAPTER 3

1. Kelly, J., 2021. What is Diabetes?. [online] Cdc.gov. Available at: <https://www.cdc.gov/media/presskits/aahd/diabetes.pdf> [Accessed 4 May 2021].
2. National Center for Biotechnology Information. 2010. Diagnosis and Classification of Diabetes Mellitus. [online] Available at: <https://www.ncbi.nlm.nih.gov/pmc/articles/PMC2797383/> [Accessed 4 May 2021].
3. Weatherspoon D. History of diabetes: early science, early treatment, insulin [Internet]. Medical News Today. MediLexicon International; 2007 [cited 2021May7]. Available from: https://www.medicalnewstoday.com/articles/317484
4. Mayo Clinic Staff. Hyperglycemia in diabetes [Internet]. Mayo Clinic. Mayo Foundation for Medical Education and Research; 2020 [cited 2021May8]. Available from: https://www.mayoclinic.org/diseases-conditions/hyperglycemia/symptoms-causes/syc-20 373631#:~:text=High%20blood%20sugar%20(hyperglycemia)%20affects,taking%20eno ugh%20glucose%2Dlowering%20medication.
5. Brownlee M. The Pathobiology of Diabetic Complications [Internet]. Diabetes. American Diabetes Association; 2005 [cited 2021May7]. Available from: https://diabetes.diabetesjournals.org/content/54/6/1615#:~:text=The%20answer%20is%2 0that%20most,efficiently%20(3%2C4).
6. Glycogenolysis [Internet]. Encyclopædia Britannica. Encyclopædia Britannica, inc.; 2016 [cited 2021May7]. Available from: https://www.britannica.com/science/glycogenolysis
7. Gastaldelli A, Gaggini M, DeFronzo RA. Role of Adipose Tissue Insulin Resistance in the Natural History of Type 2 Diabetes: Results From the San Antonio Metabolism Study [Internet]. Diabetes. American Diabetes Association; 2017 [cited 2021May7]. Available from: https://diabetes.diabetesjournals.org/content/66/4/815#:~:text=Insulin%20acts%20on%20 adipose%20tissue,circulation%20(6%2C7)
8. Röder PV, Wu B, Liu Y, Han W. Pancreatic regulation of glucose homeostasis [Internet]. Experimental & molecular medicine. Nature Publishing Group; 2016 [cited 2021May7]. Available from: https://www.ncbi.nlm.nih.gov/pmc/articles/PMC4892884/
9. OpenStax LL&. Anatomy and Physiology II [Internet]. Lumen. 2021 [cited 2021May7]. Available from: https://courses.lumenlearning.com/ap2/chapter/the-endocrine-pancreas/#:~:text=Glucose %20is%20required%20for%20cellular,fuel%20for%20all%20body%20cells.&text=Rece ptors%20

located%20in%20the%20pancreas,insulin%20to%20maintain%20nor-mal%20le vels

10. OpenStax LL&. Anatomy and Physiology II [Internet]. Lumen. 2021 [cited 2021May7]. Available from: https://courses.lumenlearning.com/ap2/chapter/the-endocrine-pancreas/#:~:text=Glucose %20is%20required%20for%20cellular,fuel%20for%20all%20body%20cells.&text=Rece ptors%20located%20in%20the%20pancreas,insulin%20to%20maintain%20nor-mal%20le vels

11. Choo SY. The HLA System: Genetics, Immunology, Clinical Testing, and Clinical Implications [Internet]. The National Center for Biotechnology Information. Yonsei Medical Journal; 2007 [cited 2021May7]. Available from: https://www.ncbi.nlm.nih.gov/pmc/articles/PMC2628004/

12. Noble JA, Valdes AM. Genetics of the HLA region in the prediction of type 1 diabetes [Internet]. Current diabetes reports. U.S. National Library of Medicine; 2011 [cited 2021May7]. Available from: https://www.ncbi.nlm.nih.gov/pmc/articles/PMC3233362/#:~:text=Type%201%20diabete s%20(T1D)%20is,genes%20encoding%20DQ%20and%20DR.

13. Saberzadeh-Ardestani B, Karamzadeh R, Basiri M, Hajizadeh-Saffar E, Farhadi A, Shapiro AMJ, et al. Type 1 Diabetes Mellitus: Cellular and Molecular Pathophysiology at A Glance [Internet]. Cell journal. Royan Institute; 2018 [cited 2021May7]. Available from: https://www.ncbi.nlm.nih.gov/pmc/articles/PMC6004986/

14. Dabelea D, D'Agostino RB, Mayer-Davis EJ, Pettitt DJ, Imperatore G, Dolan LM, et al. Testing the Accelerator Hypothesis [Internet]. Diabetes Care. American Diabetes Association; 2006 [cited 2021May7]. Available from: https://care.diabetesjournals.org/content/29/2/290

15. CA; D. Proinflammatory cytokines [Internet]. Chest. U.S. National Library of Medicine; 2000 [cited 2021May7]. Available from: https://pubmed.ncbi.nlm.nih.gov/10936147/#:~:text=Results%3A%20Cytokines%20are %20regulators%20of,healing%20(anti%2Dinflammatory)

16. Basu R. Type 1 Diabetes [Internet]. National Institute of Diabetes and Digestive and Kidney Diseases. U.S. Department of Health and Human Services; 2017 [cited 2021May7]. Available from: https://www.niddk.nih.gov/health-information/diabetes/overview/what-is-diabetes/type-1 -diabetes

17. Delves PJ. Human Leukocyte Antigen (HLA) System - Immunology; Allergic Disorders [Internet]. Merck Manuals Professional Edition. Merck Manuals; 2020 [cited 2021May8]. Available from: https://www.merckmanuals.com/en-ca/professional/immunology-allergic-disorders/biolo gy-of-the-immune-system/human-leukocyte-antigen-hla-system#:~:text=The%20human %20leukocyte%20antigen%20

18. American Diabetes Association. 2. Classification and Diagnosis of Diabetes [Internet]. Diabetes Care. American Diabetes Association; 2015 [cited 2021May8]. Available from: https://care.diabetesjournals.org/content/38/Supplement_1/S8

19. Cai S, Fu X, Sheng Z. Dedifferentiation: A New Approach in Stem Cell Research [Internet]. OUP Academic. Oxford University Press; 2007 [cited 2021May8]. Available from: https://academic.oup.com/bioscience/article/57/8/655/284571

20. Cerf ME. Beta cell dysfunction and insulin resistance [Internet]. Frontiers in endocrinology. Frontiers Media S.A.; 2013 [cited 2021May8]. Available from: https://www.ncbi.nlm.nih.gov/pmc/articles/PMC3608918/#:~:text=Beta%20cell%20dysf unction%20results%20from,in%20the%20 manifestation%20of%20hyperglycemia.

21. Lillis C. Insulin sensitivity: How to improve it naturally [Internet]. Medical News Today. MediLexicon International; 2019 [cited 2021May8]. Available from: https://www.medicalnewstoday.com/articles/323027

22. Plows JF, Stanley JL, Baker PN, Reynolds CM, Vickers MH. The Pathophysiology of Gestational Diabetes Mellitus [Internet]. International journal of molecular sciences. MDPI; 2018 [cited 2021May8]. Available from: https://www.ncbi.nlm.nih.gov/pmc/articles/PMC6274679/#:~:text=%CE%B2%2Dcell%2 0dysfunction%20is%20exacerbated,described%20 as%20glucotoxicity%20%5B76%5D.

23. Nationwide Children's Hospital. Diabetes: MODY [Internet]. Diabetes MODY: Causes, Symptoms, Diagnosis and Treatment. 2020 [cited 2021May8]. Available from: https://www.nationwidechildrens.org/conditions/diabetes-mody

24. How insulin works [Internet]. YouTube. YouTube; 2018 [cited 2021May8]. Available from: https://www.youtube.com/watch?v=HJGjNT-Jgf48

25. The Role of Insulin in the Human Body [Internet]. YouTube. YouTube; 2011 [cited 2021May8]. Available from: https://www.youtube.com/watch?v=OYH1deu7-4E

26. Dansinger M. Type 1 Diabetes: Causes, Symptoms, Treatments, Diagnosis, and PreventionM [Internet]. WebMD. WebMD; 2019 [cited 2021May8]. Available from: https://www.webmd.com/diabetes/type-1-diabetes#:~:text=Type%201%20diabetes%20is %20a,to%20be%20called%20 juvenile%20diabetes.

27. Cantley J, Ashcroft FM. Q&A: insulin secretion and type 2 diabetes: why do β-cells fail? [Internet]. BMC biology. BioMed Central; 2015 [cited 2021May8]. Available from: https://www.ncbi.nlm.nih.gov/pmc/articles/PMC4435650/#CR2

CHAPTER 4

1. Baeres FMM, Gundgaard J, Brown-Frandsen K. What is innovation in the area of medicines? The example of insulin and diabetes. Diabetic Medicine [Internet]. 2019 Dec 1;36(12):1528–9. Available from:http://resolver.

scholarsportal.info.libaccess.lib.mcmaster.ca/resolve/07423071/v36i0 012/1528_wiiitateoiad.xml

2. Biscontini T. Insulin. Salem Press Encyclopedia of Health [Internet]. 2019 [cited 2021 May 4]; Available from: http://search.ebscohost.com.libaccess.lib.mcmaster.ca/login.aspx?direct=true&db=ers&AN=93788032&site=eds-live&scope=site

3. Catalano PM. Obesity, insulin resistance and pregnancy outcome. Reproduction (Cambridge, England). 2010 Sep;140(3):365.

4. Chantelau E., Lee D. M., Hemmann D. M., Zipfel U., Echterhoff S. What Makes Insulin Injections Painful? BMJ: British Medical Journal [Internet]. 1991 Jul 6 [cited 2021 May 4];303(6793):26–7. Available from: http://search.ebscohost.com.libaccess.lib.mcmaster.ca/login.aspx?direct=true&db=edsjsr &AN=edsjsr.29712186&site=eds-live&scope=site

5. Kelley DE. Overview: what is insulin resistance? Nutrition reviews [Internet]. 2000 Mar [cited 2021 May 4];58(3 Pt 2):S2–3. Available from: http://search.ebscohost.com.libaccess.lib.mcmaster.ca/login.aspx?direct=true&db=cmed m&AN=10812925&site=eds-live&scope=site

6. Lambert, K. and Holt, R.I.G. (2013), The use of insulin analogues in pregnancy. Diabetes Obes Metab, 15: 888-900. https://doi.org/10.1111/dom.12098

7. Michael D. Insulin Resistance [Internet]. WebMD. 2019 [cited 3 May 2021]. Available from: https://www.webmd.com/diabetes/insulin-resistance-syndrome

8. Reading: Protein Structure | Biology I [Internet]. Courses.lumenlearning.com. [cited 4 May 2021]. Available from: https://courses.lumenlearning.com/ivytech-bio1- 1/chapter/reading-protein-structure/

9. Types of Insulin [Internet]. HealthLink BC. 2019 [cited 3 May 2021]. Available from: https://www.healthlinkbc.ca/health-topics/aa122570

10. Vargas E, Joy NV, Sepulveda MA. Biochemistry, Insulin Metabolic Effects. StatPearls [Internet]. 2020 Mar 28.)

11. Wilcox G. Insulin and Insulin Resistance [Internet]. PubMed Central (PMC). 2005 [cited 4 May 2021]. Available from: https://www.ncbi.nlm.nih.gov/pmc/articles/PMC1204764

CHAPTER 5

1. Russell-Jones D, Pouwer F, Khunti K. Identification of barriers to insulin therapy and approaches to overcoming them. Diabetes Obes Metab. 2018 Mar;20(3):488-496. doi: 10.1111/dom.13132.

2. Ory MG, Lee S, Towne SD Jr., Flores S, Gabriel O, Smith ML. Implementing a Diabetes Education Program to Reduce Health Disparities in South Texas: Application of the RE-AIM Framework for Planning and Evaluation.

International Journal of Environmental Research and Public Health. 2020; 17(17):6312. https://doi.org/10.3390/ijerph17176312

3. Titus SK, Kataoka-Yahiro M. Barriers to Access to Care in Hispanics With Type 2 Diabetes: A Systematic Review. Hispanic Health Care International. October 2020. doi:10.1177/1540415320956389

4. Karter, Andrew J., et al. Barriers to insulin initiation: the translating research into action for diabetes insulin starts project. Diabetes Care. 2010; 33(4):733. Gale Academic OneFile, link.gale.com/apps/doc/A224405302/ AONE?u=otta77973&sid=AONE&xid=af26c1f7.

5. Swaminathan K, Vinaykumar M, Cohen O. Breaking Socioeconomic Barriers in Diabetes Technologies: Outcomes of a Pilot Insulin Pump Programme for the Underprivileged in Rural India. Indian journal of endocrinology and metabolism, 2019, 23(2): 242–245.

6. Roberta, H. M., Struck, L., & Burshell, A. (2001). Empowerment for diabetes management: Integrating true self-management into the medical treatment and management of diabetes mellitus. The Ochsner Journal, 3(3), 149-157. Retrieved from https://login.proxy.bib.uottawa.ca/login?url=https:// www-proquest-com.proxy.bib.uottaw a.ca/scholarly-journals/empowerment-diabetes-management-integrating-true/docview/21 57906387/se-2?accountid=14701

CHAPTER 6

1. Mayfield JA, White RD. Insulin therapy for type 2 diabetes: rescue, augmentation, and replacement of beta-cell function. Am Fam Physician. 2004 Aug 1;70(3):489-500. Erratum in: Am Fam Physician. 2004 Dec 1;70(11):2079-80. PMID: 15317436.

2. Nathan DM. The Diabetes Control and Complications Trial/Epidemiology of Diabetes Interventions and Complications Study at 30 Years: Overview. Diabetes Care Jan 2014, 37 (1) 9-16; DOI: 10.2337/dc13-2112

3. UK Prospective Diabetes Study (UKPDS) Group Intensive blood-glucose control with sulphonylureas or insulin compared with conventional treatment and risk of complications in patients with type 2 diabetes (UKPDS 33) Lancet. 1998;352:837–853. doi: 10.1016/S0140-6736(98)07019-6.

4. Kitzmiller JL, Gavin LA, Gin GD, Jovanovic-Peterson L, Main EK, Zigrang WD. Preconception Care of Diabetes: Glycemic Control Prevents Congenital Anomalies. JAMA. 1991;265(6):731–736. doi:10.1001/ jama.1991.03460060063025

5. Turok DK, Ratcliffe SD, Baxley EG. Management of gestational diabetes mellitus. Am Fam Physician. 2003 Nov 1;68(9):1767-72. Erratum in: Am Fam Physician. 2004 Mar 15;69(6):1362. PMID: 14620596.

6. Kineman RD, Del Rio-Moreno M, Sarmento-Cabral A. 40 YEARS of IGF1: Understanding the tissue-specific roles of IGF1/IGF1R in reg-

ulating metabolism using the Cre/loxP system. J Mol Endocrinol (2018) 61(1):T187–98. doi: 10.1530/JME-18-0076

7. Mohamed-Ali V, Pinkney J. Therapeutic potential of insulin-like growth factor-1 in patients with diabetes mellitus. Treat Endocrinol. 2002;1(6):399-410. doi: 10.2165/00024677-200201060-00005. PMID: 15832492.

8. Wilcox G. Insulin and insulin resistance. Clin Biochem Rev. 2005;26(2):19-39

CHAPTER 7

1. Oleck J, Kassam S, Goldman JD. Commentary: Why Was Inhaled Insulin a Failure in the Market? Diabetes Spectrum. 2016;29(3):180–4.

2. Madhu SV, Velmurugan M. Future of newer basal insulin. Indian Journal of Endocrinology and Metabolism. 2013;17(2):249.

3. Iyer H, Khedkar A, Verma M. Oral insulin - a review of current status. Diabetes, Obesity and Metabolism. 2010;12(3):179–85.

4. Bernstein G. Delivery of insulin to the buccal mucosa utilizing the RapidMist™ system. Expert Opinion on Drug Delivery. 2008;5(9):1047–55.

5. Zhang Y, Yu J, Kahkoska AR, Wang J, Buse JB, Gu Z. Advances in transdermal insulin delivery. Advanced Drug Delivery Reviews. 2019;139:51–70.

6. Insulin Administration. Diabetes Care. 2003;26(1).

7. Shah RB, Shah VN, Patel M, Maahs DM. Insulin delivery methods: Past, present and future. International Journal of Pharmaceutical Investigation. 2016;6(1):1.

8. Freude S, Plum L, Schnitker J, Leeser U, Udelhoven M, Krone W, et al. Peripheral Hyperinsulinemia Promotes Tau Phosphorylation In Vivo. Diabetes. 2005;54(12):3343–8.

9. Stadler M, Anderwald C, Pacini G, Zbyn S, Promintzer-Schifferl M, Mandl M, et al. Chronic Peripheral Hyperinsulinemia in Type 1 Diabetic Patients After Successful Combined Pancreas-Kidney Transplantation Does Not Affect Ectopic Lipid Accumulation in Skeletal Muscle and Liver. Diabetes. 2009;59(1):215–8.

10. Selam J-L. Evolution of Diabetes Insulin Delivery Devices. Journal of Diabetes Science and Technology. 2010;4(3):505–13.

11. Fry A. Insulin Delivery Device Technology 2012: Where are We after 90 Years? Journal of Diabetes Science and Technology. 2012;6(4):947–53.

12. Cobden D, Lee WC, Balu S, Joshi AV, Pashos CL. Health Outcomes and Economic Impact of Therapy Conversion to a Biphasic Insulin Analog Pen Among Privately Insured Patients with Type 2 Diabetes Mellitus. Pharmacotherapy. 2007;27(7):948–62.

13. Rubin RR, Peyrot M. Quality of Life, Treatment Satisfaction, and Treatment Preference Associated With Use of a Pen Device Delivering a Premixed 70/30 Insulin Aspart Suspension (Aspart Protamine Suspension/

Soluble Aspart) Versus Alternative Treatment Strategies. Diabetes Care. 2004;27(10):2495–7.

14. Wikby A, Stenström U, Andersson P-O, Hörnquist JO. Metabolic Control, Quality of Life, and Negative Life Events: A Longitudinal Study of Well-Controlled and Poorly Regulated Patients With Type 1 Diabetes After Changeover to Insulin Pen Treatment. The Diabetes Educator. 1998;24(1):61–6.

15. Berget C, Messer LH, Forlenza GP. A Clinical Overview of Insulin Pump Therapy for the Management of Diabetes: Past, Present, and Future of Intensive Therapy. Diabetes Spectrum. 2019;32(3):194–204.

16. Retnakaran R, Zinman B. Continuous Subcutaneous Insulin Infusion Versus Multiple Daily Injections: The Impact of Baseline A1c: Response to Blumer. Diabetes Care. 2005;28(3):763–4.

17. Rask-Madsen C, King GL. Vascular Complications of Diabetes: Mechanisms of Injury and Protective Factors. Cell Metabolism. 2013;17(1):20–33.

18. Cohen O, Körner A, Chlup R, Zoupas CS, Ragozin AK, Wudi K, et al. Improved Glycemic Control through Continuous Glucose Sensor-Augmented Insulin Pump Therapy: Prospective Results from a Community and Academic Practice Patient Registry. Journal of Diabetes Science and Technology. 2009;3(4):804–11.

19. Chen E, King F, Kohn MA, Spanakis EK, Breton M, Klonoff DC. A Review of Predictive Low Glucose Suspend and Its Effectiveness in Preventing Nocturnal Hypoglycemia. Diabetes Technology & Therapeutics. 2019;21(10):602–9.

20. Rini CJ, McVey E, Sutter D, Keith S, Kurth H-J, Nosek L, et al. Intradermal insulin infusion achieves faster insulin action than subcutaneous infusion for 3-day wear. Drug Delivery and Translational Research. 2015;5(4):332–45.

21. Hollander PA, Blonde L, Rowe R, Mehta AE, Milburn JL, Hershon KS, et al. Efficacy and Safety of Inhaled Insulin (Exubera) Compared With Subcutaneous Insulin Therapy in Patients With Type 2 Diabetes: Results of a 6-month, randomized, comparative trial. Diabetes Care. 2004;27(10):2356–62.

22. Quattrin T, Belanger A, Bohannon NJV, Schwartz SL. Efficacy and Safety of Inhaled Insulin (Exubera) Compared With Subcutaneous Insulin Therapy in Patients With Type 1 Diabetes: Results of a 6-month, randomized, comparative trial. Diabetes Care. 2004;27(11):2622–7.

23. Fabbri L. Pulmonary safety of inhaled insulins: a review of the current data. Current Medical Research and Opinion. 2006;22(sup3).

24. Wajchenberg BL. β-Cell Failure in Diabetes and Preservation by Clinical Treatment. Endocrine Reviews. 2007;28(2):187–218.

25. Brown RJ, Rother KI. Effects of beta-cell rest on beta-cell function: a review of clinical and preclinical data. Pediatric Diabetes. 2008;9(3pt2):14–22.

26. Shechter Y, Mironchik M, Rubinraut S, Tsubery H, Sasson K, Marcus Y, et al. Reversible pegylation of insulin facilitates its prolonged action in vivo. European Journal of Pharmaceutics and Biopharmaceutics. 2008;70(1):19–28.

27. Palin KJ, Phillips AJ, Ning A. The oral absorption of cefoxitin from oil and emulsion vehicles in rats. International Journal of Pharmaceutics. 1986;33(1-3):99–104.

28. Volpatti LR, Facklam AL, Cortinas AB, Lu Y-C, Matranga MA, MacIsaac C, et al. Microgel encapsulated nanoparticles for glucose-responsive insulin delivery. Biomaterials. 2021;267:120458.

29. Guevara-Aguirre J, Guevara M, Saavedra J, Mihic M, Modi P. Beneficial Effects of Addition of Oral Spray Insulin (Oralin) on Insulin Secretion and Metabolic Control in Subjects with Type 2 Diabetes Mellitus Suboptimally Controlled on Oral Hypoglycemic Agents. Diabetes Technology & Therapeutics. 2004;6(1):1–8.

CHAPTER 8

1. Russell PJ, Fenton MB, Maxwell D, Haffie T, Nickle T. Biology: exploring the diversity of life. 4th ed. Toronto, Ontario: Nelson; 2019.

2. Fu Z, R. Gilbert E, Liu D. Regulation of Insulin Synthesis and Secretion and Pancreatic Beta-Cell Dysfunction in Diabetes. Current Diabetes Reviews [Internet]. 2012 [cited 2021May6];9(1):25–53. Available from: https://www.ncbi.nlm.nih.gov/pmc/articles/PMC3934755/

3. Melloul D, Marshak S, Cerasi E. Regulation of insulin gene transcription. Diabetologia. 2002;45(3):309–26.

4. Evans-Molina C, Garmey JC, Ketchum R, Brayman KL, Deng S, Mirmira RG. Glucose Regulation of Insulin Gene Transcription and Pre-mRNA Processing in Human Islets. Diabetes [Internet]. 2007 [cited 2021May6];56(3):827–35. Available from: https://www.ncbi.nlm.nih.gov/pmc/articles/PMC3705758/

5. OpenStax CNX. Figure 2 [Internet]. Lumen Learning. Pressbooks; [cited 2021May6]. Available from: https://courses.lumenlearning.com/wm-nmbiology1/chapter/reading-steps-of-translation/

6. Kaufman RJ. Beta-Cell Failure, Stress, and Type 2 Diabetes. New England Journal of Medicine. 2011;365(20):1931–3

CHAPTER 9

1. Cahn A, Miccoli R, Dardano A, Del Prato S. New forms of insulin and insulin therapies for the treatment of type 2 diabetes. Lancet Diabetes Endocrinol [Internet]. 2015;3(8):638–52. Available from: http://dx.doi.

org/10.1016/S2213-8587(15)00097-2

2. Niswender KD. Basal insulin: Physiology, pharmacology, and clinical implications. Postgrad Med. 2011;123(4):17–26.

3. Diabetes Education. Type 2 Non Insulin Therapies. 2021. p. 4–7.

4. Pernicova I, Korbonits M. Metformin-Mode of action and clinical implications for diabetes and cancer. Nat Rev Endocrinol. 2014;10(3):143–56.

5. Bailey CJ. Metformin: historical overview. Diabetologia. 2017;60(9):1566–76.

6. Flory J, Lipska K. Metformin in 2019. JAMA - J Am Med Assoc. 2019;321(19):1926–7.

7. Nanjan MJ, Mohammed M, Prashantha Kumar BR, Chandrasekar MJN. Thiazolidinediones as antidiabetic agents: A critical review. Bioorg Chem [Internet]. 2018;77:548–67. Available from: https://doi.org/10.1016/j.bioorg.2018.02.009

8. Mooradian A, Chehade J, Thurman J. The Role of Thiazolidinediones in the Treatment of Patients with Type 2 Diabetes Mellitus. 2002;1:13–20.

9. Barnett AH. Redefining the role of thiazolidinediones in the management of type 2 diabetes. Vasc Health Risk Manag. 2009;5:141–51.

10. Yaribeygi H, Maleki M, Sathyapalan T, Jamialahmadi T, Sahebkar A. Anti-inflammatory potentials of incretin-based therapies used in the management of diabetes. Life Sci [Internet]. 2020;241(December 2019):117152. Available from: https://doi.org/10.1016/j.lfs.2019.117152

11. Stonehouse AH, Darsow T, Maggs DG. Incretin-based therapies. J Diabetes. 2012;4(1):55–67.

12. Nauck MA, Meier JJ. The incretin effect in healthy individuals and those with type 2 diabetes: Physiology, pathophysiology, and response to therapeutic interventions. Lancet Diabetes Endocrinol [Internet]. 2016;4(6):525–36. Available from: http://dx.doi.org/10.1016/S2213-8587(15)00482-9

13. Affinati AH, Esfandiari NH, Oral EA, Kraftson AT. Bariatric Surgery in the Treatment of Type 2 Diabetes. Curr Diab Rep. 2019;19(12).

14. Richards et al. Diabetes after Bariatric Surgery. Physiol Behav. 2018;176(5):139–48.

15. Bekiari E, Kitsios K, Thabit H, Tauschmann M, Athanasiadou E, Karagiannis T, et al. Artificial pancreas treatment for outpatients with type 1 diabetes: Systematic review and meta-Analysis. BMJ. 2018;361.

16. Boughton CK, Hovorka R. Is an artificial pancreas (closed-loop system) for Type 1 diabetes effective? Diabet Med. 2019;36(3):279–86.

CHAPTER 10

1. Ugwu E, Ojobi J, Ndibuagu E. Misconceptions about Insulin and Barriers to Insulin Initiation in Type 2 Diabetes among General Physicians in South-

east Nigeria. Journal of Advances in Medicine and Medical Research. 2020 Jun 22;30–8.

2. Abu Hassan H, Tohid H, Mohd Amin R, Long Bidin MB, Muthupalaniappen L, Omar K. Factors influencing insulin acceptance among type 2 diabetes mellitus patients in a primary care clinic: a qualitative exploration. BMC Fam Pract. 2013 Dec;14(1):164.

3. Benroubi M. Fear, guilt feelings and misconceptions: Barriers to effective insulin treatment in type 2 diabetes. Diabetes Research and Clinical Practice. 2011 Aug 1;93:S97–9.

4. Wild D, von Maltzahn R, Brohan E, Christensen T, Clauson P, Gonder-Frederick L. A critical review of the literature on fear of hypoglycemia in diabetes: Implications for diabetes management and patient education. Patient Education and Counseling. 2007 Sep 1;68(1):10–5.

5. Frier BM, Jensen MM, Chubb BD. Hypoglycaemia in adults with insulin-treated diabetes in the UK: self-reported frequency and effects. Diabetic Medicine. 2016;33(8):1125–32.

6. Brunelle RL, Llewelyn J, Anderson JH, Gale EA, Koivisto VA. Meta-analysis of the effect of insulin lispro on severe hypoglycemia in patients with type 1 diabetes [Internet]. Database of Abstracts of Reviews of Effects (DARE): Quality-assessed Reviews [Internet]. Centre for Reviews and Dissemination (UK); 1998 [cited 2021 May 8]. Available from: https://www.ncbi.nlm.nih.gov/books/NBK67235/

7. Wilde MI, McTavish D. Insulin Lispro. Drugs. 1997 Oct 1;54(4):597–614.

8. Mak RH. Insulin and its role in chronic kidney disease. Pediatr Nephrol. 2008 Mar 1;23(3):355–62.

9. De Cosmo S, Menzaghi C, Prudente S, Trischitta V. Role of insulin resistance in kidney dysfunction: insights into the mechanism and epidemiological evidence. Nephrology Dialysis Transplantation. 2013 Jan 1;28(1):29–36.

10. Townsend RR. Angiotensin and insulin resistance: Conspiracy theory. Current Science Inc. 2003 Apr 1;5(2):110–6.

11. Lastra-Lastra G, Sowers JR, Restrepo-Erazo K, Manrique-Acevedo C, Lastra-González G. Role of aldosterone and angiotensin II in insulin resistance: an update. Clinical Endocrinology. 2009;71(1):1–6.

12. Ogihara Takehide, Asano Tomoichiro, Ando Katsuyuki, Chiba Yuko, Sakoda Hideyuki, Anai Motonobu, et al. Angiotensin II–Induced Insulin Resistance Is Associated With Enhanced Insulin Signaling. Hypertension. 2002 Dec 1;40(6):872–9.

13. Olivares-Reyes JA, Arellano-Plancarte A, Castillo-Hernandez JR. Angiotensin II and the development of insulin resistance: Implications for diabetes. Molecular and Cellular Endocrinology. 2009 Apr 29;302(2):128–39.

14. Folli F, Saad MJ, Velloso L, Hansen H, Carandente O, Feener EP, et al. Crosstalk between insulin and angiotensin II signalling systems. Exp Clin Endocrinol Diabetes. 1999;107(2):133–9.

15. Henriksen Erik J., Jacob Stephan, Kinnick Tyson R., Teachey Mary K., Krekler Michael. Selective Angiotensin II Receptor Antagonism Reduces Insulin Resistance in Obese Zucker Rats. Hypertension. 2001 Oct 1;38(4):884–90.

16. Swiderska E, Strycharz J, Wróblewski A, Szemraj J, Drzewoski J, Śliwińska A. Role of PI3K/AKT Pathway in Insulin-Mediated Glucose Uptake. In 2018.

17. Brod M, Alolga SL, Meneghini L. Barriers to Initiating Insulin in Type 2 Diabetes Patients: Development of a New Patient Education Tool to Address Myths, Misconceptions and Clinical Realities. Patient. 2014 Dec 1;7(4):437–50.

CHAPTER 11

1. Chaudhari N, & Roper SD. The cell biology of taste. J Cell Biol. 2010; 190(3):285-296.

2. Busque SM, Kerstetter JE, Geibel JP, and Insogna K. L-type amino acids stimulate gastric acid secretion by activation of the calcium-sensing receptor in parietal cells. Am J Physiol Gastrointest Liver Physiol. 2005; 289(4):G664-G669.

3. Fábián TK, Beck A, Fejérdy P, Hermann P, & Fábián G. Molecular Mechanisms of Taste Recognition: Considerations about the Role of Saliva. Int J Mol Sci. 2015; 16:5945-5974.

4. Furness JB, Rivera LR, Cho H, Bravo DM, & Callaghan B. The gut as a sensory organ. Nat Rev Gastroenterol Hepatol. 2013; 10:729-740.

5. Horio N, Yoshida R, Yasumatsu K, Yanagawa Y, Ishimaru Y, Matsunami H, & Ninomiya Y. Sour Taste Responses in Mice Lacking PKD Channels. PLoS ONE. 2011; 6(5): e20007.

6. Kinnamon SC, & Vandenbeuch A. Receptors and transduction of umami taste stimuli. Ann N Y Acad Sci. 2009; 1170:55-59.

7. Kojima I, & Nakagawa Y. The Role of the Sweet Taste Receptor in Enteroendocrine Cells and Pancreatic β-Cells. Diabetes Metab J. 2011; 35:451-457.

8. Lee CW, Rivera R, Gardell S, Dubin AE, & Chun J. GPR92 as a new G12/13- and Gq-coupled lysophosphatidic acid receptor that increases cAMP, LPA5. J Biol Chem. 2006; 281(33):23589-23597.

9. Margolskee RF. Molecular Mechanisms of Bitter and Sweet Taste Transduction. J Biol Chem. 2002; 277:1-4.

10. Nakamura E, Uneyama H, & Torii K. Gastrointestinal nutrient chemosensing and the gut-brain axis: Significance of glutamate signaling for normal digestion. J Gastroenterol Hepatol. 2013; 28(S4): 2-8.

11. Nguyen CA, Akiba Y, & Kaunitz JD. Recent advances in gut nutrient chemosensing. Curr Med Chem. 2012; 19(1): 28-34.

100

12. Psichas A, Page AJ, Martin CM, & Blackshaw LA. Vagal Mechanoreceptors and Chemoreceptors in Mouse Stomach and Esophagus. J Neurosci. 2002; 87(4): 2095-2103.

13. Raybould H. Gut Chemosensing: Interactions between Gut Endocrine Cells and Visceral Afferents. Auton Neurosci. 2010; 153(1-2): 41–46.

14. Reimann F, & Gribble FM. Gut chemosensing mechanisms. J Clin Invest. 2015; 125(3): 908–917.

15. Rettenberger AT, Schulze W, Breer H, & Haid D. Analysis of the protein related receptor GPR92 in G-cells. Front Physiol. 2015; 261(6): 1-8.

16. Richter TA, Dvoriyanchikov GA, Roper SD, & Chaudari N. Acid-Sensing Ion Channel-2 Is Not Necessary for Sour Taste in Mice. J Neurosci. 2004; 4(16):4088 – 4091.

17. Sbarbati A, Merigo F, Benati D, Tizzano M, Bernardi P, & Osculati F. Laryngeal chemosensory clusters. Chem Senses. 2004; 29 (8): 683-692.

18. Sternini C, Anselmi L, & Rozengurt E. Enteroendocrine cells: a site of "taste" in gastrointestinal chemosensing. Curr Opin Endocrinol Diabetes Obes. 2008; 15(1):73-78.

19. Cernea, S., & Raz, I. (2019). Insulin Therapy: Future Perspectives. American Journal of Therapeutics, 1. doi:10.1097/mjt.0000000000001076

20. McGill, J. B., Peters, A., Buse, J. B., Steiner, S., Tran, T., Pompilio, F. M., & Kendall, D. M. (2020). Comprehensive Pulmonary Safety Review of Inhaled Technosphere® Insulin in Patients with Diabetes Mellitus. Clinical drug investigation, 40(10), 973–983. https://doi.org/10.1007/s40261-020-00958-8

www.ingramcontent.com/pod-product-compliance
Lightning Source LLC
Chambersburg PA
CBHW022103210326
41518CB00039B/781